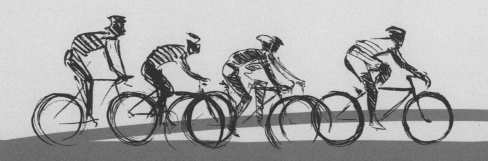

the
cyclingchef

BLOOMSBURY SPORT
Bloomsbury Publishing Plc
50 Bedford Square, London, WC1B 3DP, UK
29 Earlsfort Terrace, Dublin 2, Ireland

BLOOMSBURY, BLOOMSBURY SPORT and the Diana logo are trademarks of Bloomsbury Publishing Plc

First published in Great Britain in 2019

Food photography by Clare Winfield
Food styling by Rebecca Woods
Other photography by Grant Pritchard
Design by Sian Rance for D.R. ink

Images on pp. 8–9, 22–3, 26, 38–9, 52, 62–3, 98, 110, 134, 136, 144, 146, 160, 162, 182 and 184 © Getty Images

British Library Cataloguing-in-Publication Data

A catalogue record for this book is available from the British Library

Library of Congress Cataloguing-in-Publication data has been applied for

ISBN: HB: 978-1-4729-6002-3; ePDF: 978-1-4729-6000-9; ePub: 978-1-4729-6003-0

6 8 10 9 7 5

Typeset in ITC Century by D.R. ink
Printed and bound in Great Britain by Bell and Bain Ltd, Glasgow

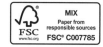

Bloomsbury Publishing Plc makes every effort to ensure that the papers used in the manufacture of our books are natural, recyclable products made from wood grown in well-managed forests. Our manufacturing processes conform to the environmental regulations of the country of origin.

To find out more about our authors and books visit www.bloomsbury.com and sign up for our newsletters

ALAN MURCHISON

the cyclingchef

RECIPES FOR PERFORMANCE AND PLEASURE

BLOOMSBURY SPORT

LONDON · OXFORD · NEW YORK · NEW DELHI · SYDNEY

Contents

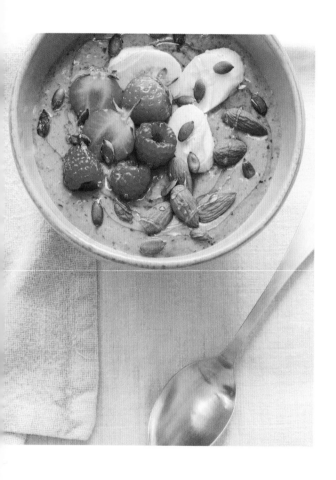

Breakfasts

Broths and Soups

Main Meals

Smoothies and Snacks

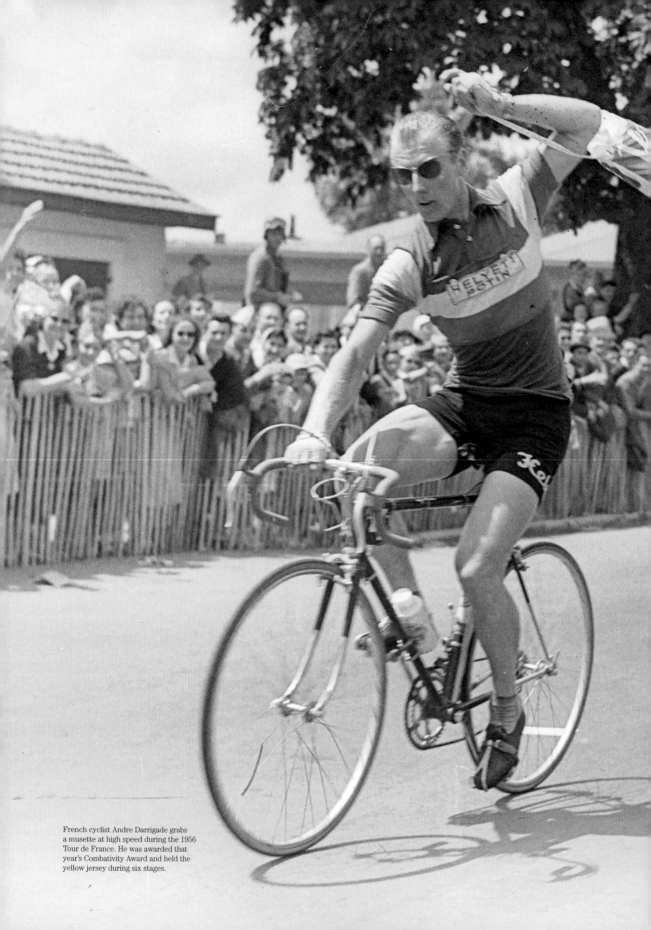

French cyclist Andre Darrigade grabs a musette at high speed during the 1956 Tour de France. He was awarded that year's Combativity Award and held the yellow jersey during six stages.

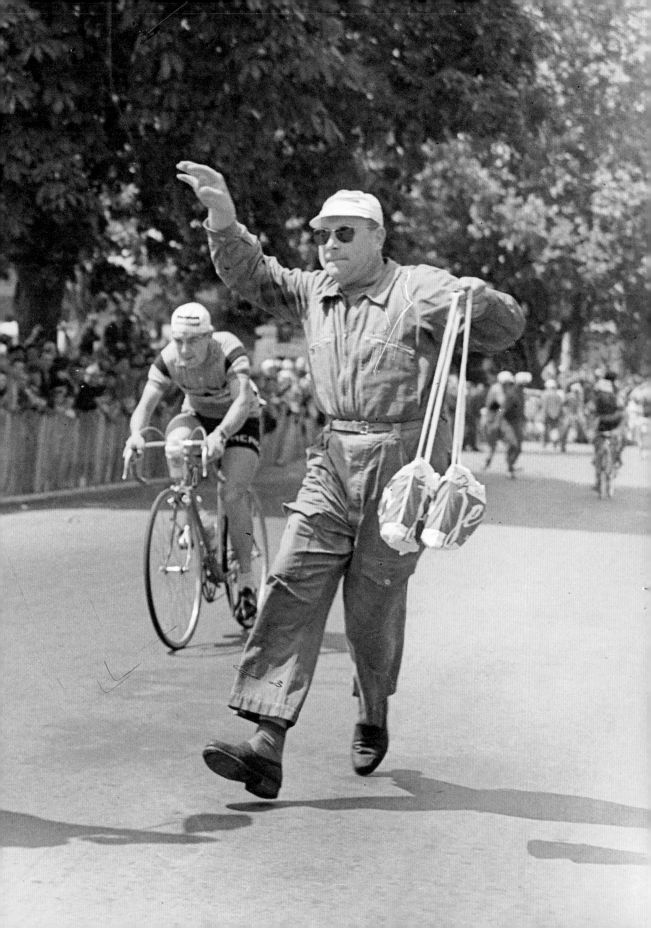

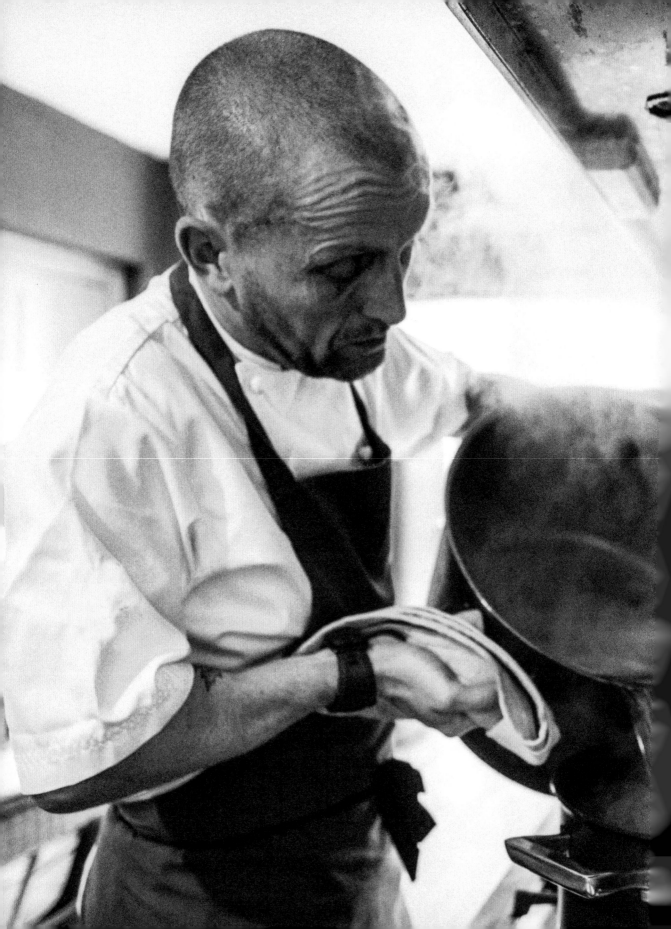

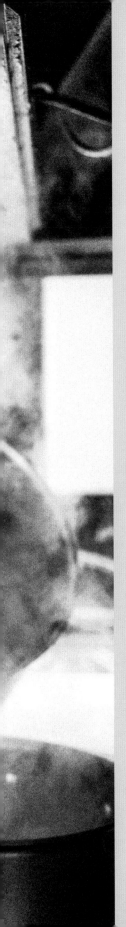

Introduction

Cycling and food are the twin passions of my life. In Performance Chef, the business I set up in 2016 to provide meal planning, recovery strategies and race fuelling advice to elite athletes, I'm able to combine my experience as a Michelin-starred restaurant chef with a first-hand knowledge of elite sport. The guiding philosophy of Performance Chef is that nutrition is not only an integral part of any athlete's planning and preparation, but also that food should satisfy the appetite and the taste buds: food that is both for pleasure and for performance.

One constant I see on a daily basis is that the quality of the food they eat and a well-balanced diet are key to their improvement, recovery and general good health.

This book gives me the opportunity to expound upon that philosophy and provide recipes that any aspiring high-performance cyclist can follow.

I'm in the fortunate position of working with cyclists of all abilities, from Olympic champions, Commonwealth medallists and World Tour riders to those who are entering their first sportive, and one constant I see on a daily basis is that the quality of the food they eat and a well-balanced diet are key to their improvement, recovery and general good health.

Athletes want – and need – to eat well to maximise their performance. However, the majority of professional or elite cyclists are training so hard that there is nothing they want to do less than spend hours in a kitchen slaving over a stove. Similarly, recreational cyclists of all abilities have limited time during the day to deal with training, work, kids, family and general living, let alone mastering complicated nutritional information. Post-ride, no cyclist ever stands in a supermarket in their bib shorts, working out the macronutrients of the food they have thrown into their shopping trolley. They want to eat, they want to train and they want to feed themselves as best they can with the limited inclination, time, knowledge or money they have at their disposal, and that's where this book can help.

If you're not training or racing as well as you had envisaged then it's probably down to over- or under-training (if you use a platform like TrainingPeaks [www.trainingpeaks.com] or are coached well, this is pretty unlikely); not recovering properly; or under- or over-fuelling. Training load must be matched with appropriate fuelling, so your food requirements will vary considerably from day to day and from month to month depending on how much you are doing.

Your daily intake will depend on your training and race schedule. You don't need a 5000-calorie day when you're doing a 60-minute recovery ride any more than you can get by drinking water and eating a green salad with some grilled chicken when you've been out for an 'honest' 100-miler. Hill reps, over-geared work, intervals or race simulation that can cause muscle damage also require high-protein and high-carbohydrate recovery meals to help refuel and repair. This demands some forethought and preparation, particularly if you're fitting your training into a working day.

Once you've accepted the link between fuelling and training and the importance of both to performance, you're halfway there. Your nutritional plans will include a balance of vegetables, grains, meat, pulses and fish, but what and when you eat will depend on your training and racing schedule. Meals can be planned in detail if that's how you roll, but items in the same food groups are often interchangeable according to what you fancy, so red meat can be swapped for chicken, kale for broccoli, kidney beans for aduki beans, etc.

As a chef in top restaurants, I've learned to have confidence in ingredients, to let food groups stand up for themselves and give meals colour, flavour and texture, but a few key skills and tips can make a real difference to how you approach cooking and eating. It isn't difficult; there's a massive choice of ingredients open to you, all easily obtainable at your local supermarket. Most of the athletes I work with have really rich and varied diets, eating food that helps improve their performance while tasting pretty good.

When I was a lad home cooking was just what you did. I cooked my first meal for my

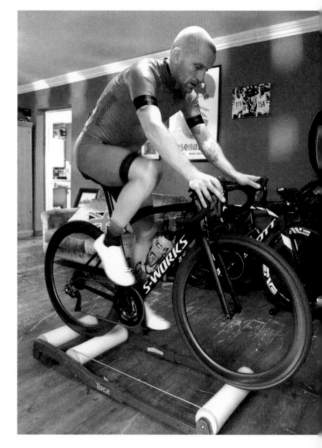

Cyclists need to eat well to maximise their performance. It is important to accept the link between fuelling and training and the importance of both to performance.

> I'm not looking to change the world, but if I can convince you to cook even one meal a day using fresh, seasonal ingredients then that's a start and your cycling will benefit from it.

family at the tender age of eight. We made everything from scratch. Bread, pancakes, sauces and soups; these food and flavour memories are deeply ingrained in me. As both my sets of grandparents lived in rural farming communities they learnt how to utilise seasonal ingredients. There was always a pot of soup on the go, breakfast was almost always based around oats as they were cheap and gave you energy for the rest of the day, and processed food was just not 'on the menu'.

Cooking three meals a day from scratch tends to be seen as a quirky kind of hobby these days. Now, I'm not looking to change the world, but if I can convince you to cook even one meal a day using fresh, seasonal ingredients then that's a start and your cycling will benefit from it. Because, as vital as your food choices are to your performance, there is one rule that supersedes all others: you must enjoy your food. It sounds obvious, but boredom, disinterest and a lack of appetite for food are your biggest enemies. Eating is not the equivalent of lubing the bike chain; it has to be a pleasure, not a chore. Food for performance, food for pleasure.

Alan Murchison, 2018

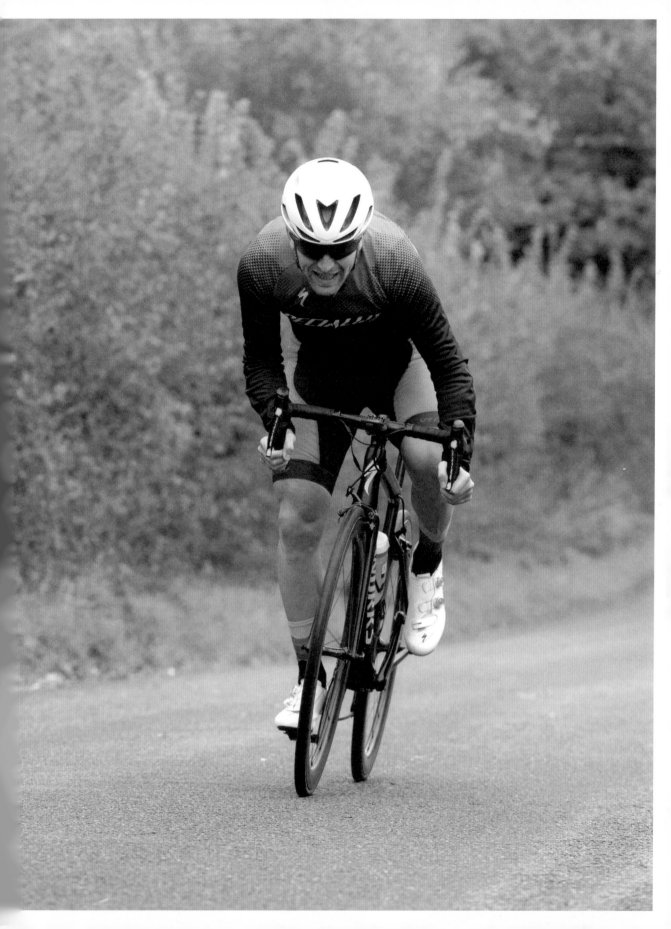

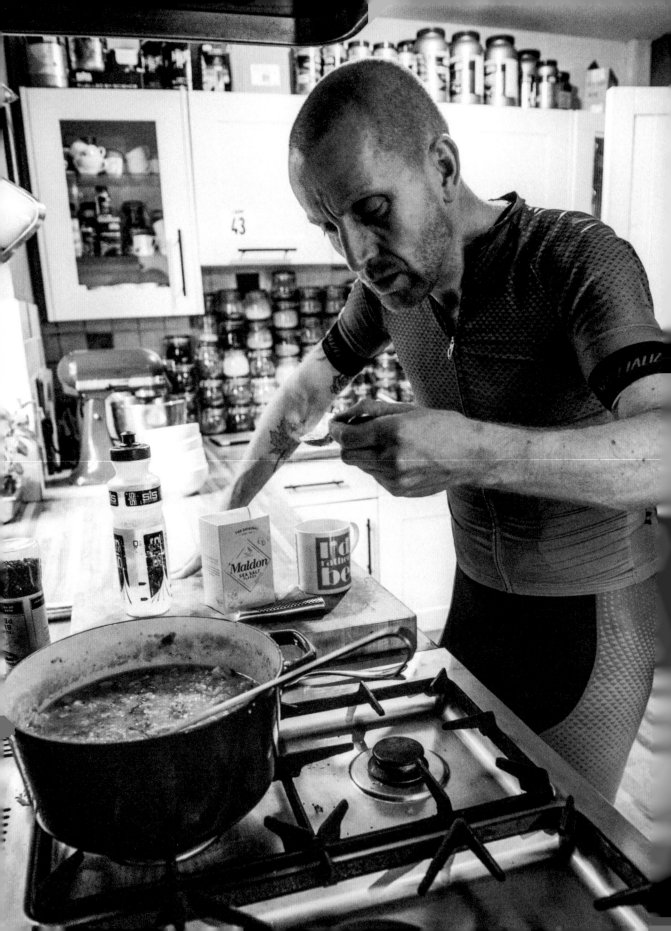

Nutritional Basics

My philosophy is pretty simple: cyclists need to eat. They need to eat well and they need to eat optimally. None of this is rocket science and much of it is down to common sense. It's about eating the foods your parents told you were good for you – vegetables, fruit, fish, grains and meat; cooking with real food – you know, the stuff that doesn't need a label; and taking advantage of great nutritional powerhouses such as chickpeas, avocados, sardines and peanut butter.

If I can convince you to cook even one meal a day using fresh, seasonal ingredients then that's a start and your cycling will benefit from it.

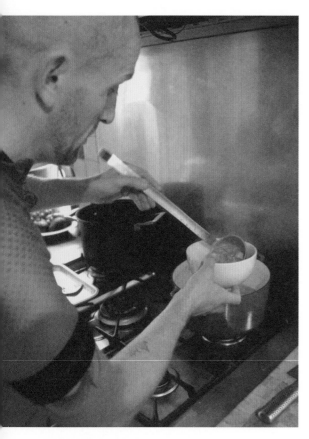

Depending on gender and training intensity, you can burn 10 calories or more a minute during a session, so it stands to reason that you need to consume more than the average person.

I'd rather not write about science. I'm much happier discussing cycling or food, but if you want to maximise your performance, it's impossible to avoid learning about how your body deals with what you eat. As a serious cyclist you're putting your body through some pretty extreme stress, and what and when you eat and drink are as vital to your numbers as your training or your bike. We tend to call it fuelling the body, but not all fuels are equal. Some are good for energy, some for muscle repair, some for well-being – and some do little good at all. It's as well to know which are which...

First of all, remember that cyclists are normal people too and your body has the same requirements as everyone else's. The World Health Organization lists these vital foods and fluids as: macronutrients, the energy sources which include proteins, carbohydrates and fats; micronutrients, the vitamins and minerals that are essential to a healthy body; and water, which makes up 60 per cent of your weight and facilitates virtually every bodily process. A balanced diet that encompasses all these gives us the muscle development, immune system, efficient body functions and energy to live an active life.

Anything we eat has a calorific value: the amount of energy present in a food. An intake of calories is essential to enable our bodies to perform tasks, and keep the heart beating and lungs operating during periods of rest. An average man requires around 2500 calories a day while a woman requires around 2000. This, of course, varies from person to person, especially for athletes, who expend more energy but whose bodies are also more efficient at creating energy. The nub of the matter is that calories can only be used or stored. If you don't consume enough calories your body will feel sluggish; too many and the body will store them in the form of fat.

As a cyclist, this is ultra-important and in terms of energy alone you immediately have some calculations to make about what you eat and when. Depending on gender and training intensity, riders can burn 10 calories or more a minute during a session, so it stands to reason that you need to consume more than the average person. Unless you're trying to lose weight (see p. 185), consuming too many calories is not a major issue for most high-performance cyclists. However, what is vital is that you consume enough calories from the right food sources.

Most of us are aware of 'evil' high-calorie foods such as chocolate, crisps, pastries, cheese and deep-fried fast foods, but some foods labelled 'healthy', such as dried fruit, nut butters and avocado, are also high in calories. However, what matters to a cyclist is the other benefits derived from these foods. Your performance will depend on maintaining an optimum weight; you require the energy to drive your body to the pain barrier; your immune system needs to be at its highest level to endure periods of immense stress and your muscles will need constant repair and growth. This is why what you eat matters more than it does to the average person – even if they are weight- and health-conscious.

When you're rolling along in the peloton, taking a light ride to stretch the legs or popping down to the shops, at low intensities your body is quite happy using fats as an energy source. It's only when you start pushing down on the pedals that things change. The harder or faster you ride, the more your body uses carbohydrates to create the energy it needs. And then, once your ride is over, your muscles will need protein to help them repair. So, in order to be fuelled efficiently, a cyclist needs to include fat, carbohydrates and protein in their diet.

As a serious cyclist you're putting your body through pretty extreme stress, and what and when you eat and drink are as vital to your numbers as your training or your bike.

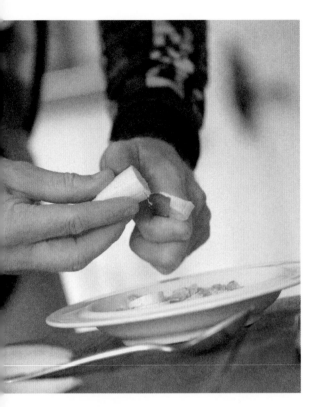

There are two forms of carbohydrate: slow-releasing and quick-releasing. While the latter is often seen as 'empty calories', there is a place for it in the cyclist's diet on occasions when quickly digestible carbs are required.

Carbohydrates

Carbohydrates are macronutrients – the primary source of, and the fastest way the body has of obtaining, energy. They derive from the sugars, starches and fibres found in fruits, grains, vegetables and dairy products.

Each carbohydrate food has a unique effect on blood glucose concentration, and many factors influence the speed at which they are digested or absorbed; for example the type and amount of fibre the food also contains, and the way in which different carbohydrates are structured. The glycaemic index ranks foods based on blood glucose response (*see also* www.glycemicindex. com for more information).

Quick-releasing carbohydrates contain one or two sugars – which raise blood glucose levels quickly. They are mainly found in sugary foods such as cakes, sweets and soft drinks; and fast foods and junk foods which contain added sugar. As they contain few other nutrients these are often seen as 'empty calories', hence the warnings associated with having too many of them in our everyday diets. There is, however, a place for these in the cyclist's diet on the occasions when quickly digestible carbohydrates are required. The most obvious example is the use of energy gels, which cyclists utilise as a quick means of replenishing carbohydrates.

Slow-releasing carbohydrates are starches comprising three or more sugars. These are not only processed more slowly, but they also contain a number of other nutrients, which gives them their 'good carbs' tag. As the body can only store around 2000 calories in glycogen (muscle fuel) it is important for a cyclist or any endurance athlete to keep their glycogen levels topped up. This is where these slow-releasing carbs come into their own.

Proteins

Protein is another of the main macronutrients. Like carbohydrate and fat, protein can be a source of energy, but its primary function is the repair and creation of body tissue. Ingested protein is broken down by the body into amino acids, which help to form the cells. However, unlike the other macronutrients, protein cannot be stored in the body. Protein synthesis (the process whereby biological cells generate new proteins) begins immediately, but only small amounts of protein can be synthesised at any one time.

Protein requirements for athletes translate to around 1.2–2 grams of protein per kilo of body weight a day. To get some idea of what this means, an egg contains around 6 grams, half a cup of cooked chickpeas 7 grams, an ounce of cheddar 6 grams and a standard chicken breast a massive 25 grams.

Cycling puts stress on the muscles and stimulates the rate of protein synthesis necessary to generate cells for muscle recovery. Also, during endurance sessions protein breakdown in the body increases, so consuming protein during a long ride can be beneficial. Therefore, recommended levels of protein intake for cyclists could be as much as twice as high as for an ordinary person, and for professional riders it could be as much as three times as high.

You can't protein-load, so you should include a small amount of protein in most meals to achieve the required levels. Any long ride should also involve some form of small mid-ride protein top-up, which could come in the form of something that's easily portable such as nuts, biltong or whey protein. Post-ride or training is a particularly key period, because your body will be crying out for protein to repair the damage to your muscles. Ideally, within 30 minutes of a ride, you should

As the body can only store around 2000 calories in glycogen, it is important for a cyclist or any endurance athlete to keep their glycogen levels topped up.

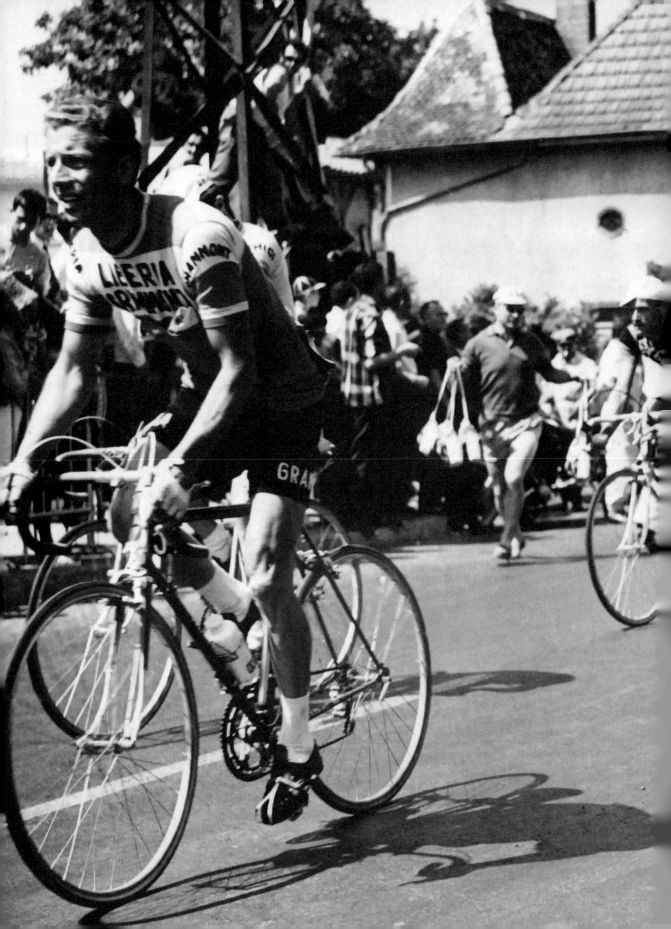

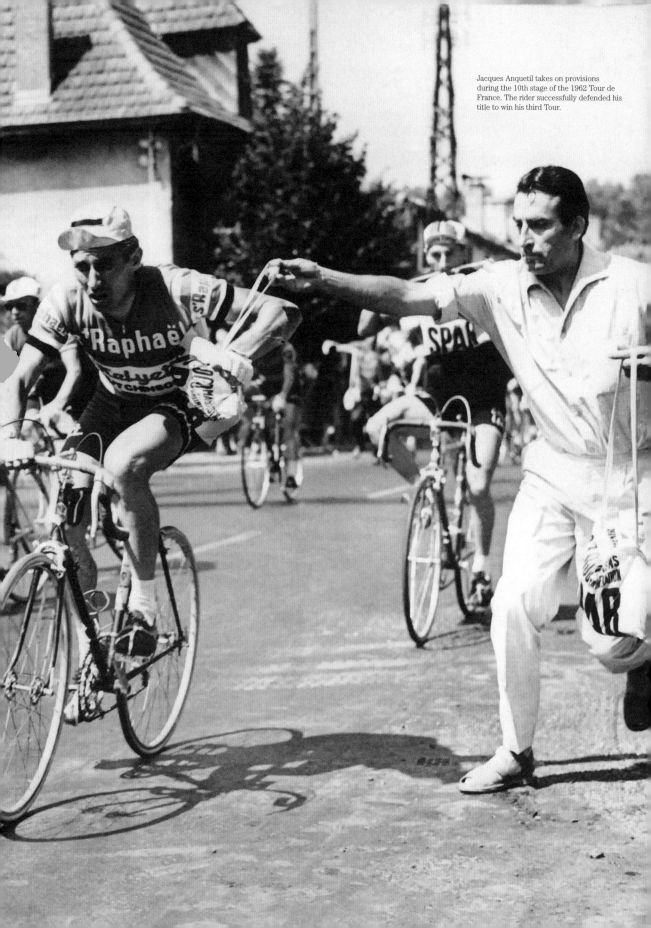

Jacques Anquetil takes on provisions
during the 10th stage of the 1962 Tour de
France. The rider successfully defended his
title to win his third Tour.

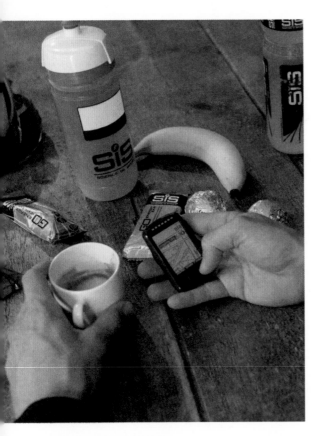

Ensuring a good nutritional intake – made up of carbohydrates, proteins, natural fats and micronutrients – will pay dividends in terms of training and racing performance.

ingest 15–25 grams of protein (around 0.3 grams per kilo of body weight) along with fast-releasing carbohydrates. Many riders choose an easily digestible smoothie with whey powder.

Fats

Third in the trio of macronutrients is fats, but what on earth can artery-clogging, cholesterol-heavy fats do for a cyclist? Fair enough. Trans-fats or hydrogenated fats can be put to one side. These are the creamy, man-made oils of crisps, biscuits and takeaways, and they are indeed good for nothing. However, natural fats do have an important role to play in a cyclist's diet.

Fats contain more than double the calories per gram of carbs or protein, so they are a way of increasing your calorie count without eating mountains of food. They also absorb vitamins A, D, E and K, aid muscle recovery and, perhaps most importantly, help bring out the flavours in food. Natural fats can be saturated and unsaturated. Butter, dairy products and palm oil are saturated fats and need to be eaten in moderation due to cholesterol issues, but unsaturated fats, such as those found in nuts and seeds, avocados and olive oil, should be an integral part of an athlete's food intake.

Particular attention should be paid to the Omega-3 fats found in oily fish, nuts, extra virgin olive oil, flax and chia seeds. These fats provide a plethora of health benefits and, of major advantage to cyclists, improve recovery by decreasing inflammation in the muscles.

Micronutrients

If macronutrients are the body's fuel, then micronutrients are the oil, because these vitamins and minerals enable the body to function effectively. Due to the demands they put on their bodies, endurance athletes need to ensure they maintain high levels of certain nutrients. It is possible to cover them all in your dietary plan, although beware of pre-packaged and processed foods, which will often have lost key nutrients in their preparation.

Among the minerals that are particularly useful to cyclists are: iron, used to build the red blood cells that carry fresh oxygen to your muscles; potassium, which regulates fluid balance, muscle contractions and nerve signals; phosphate, a mineral that helps to change protein, fat and carbohydrate into energy; magnesium, which is integral to the energy process; and calcium, another all-round vital mineral that is extra-important for strengthening cyclists' bones as these can be weakened through heavy sweating.

Sodium, a crucial mineral in the fluid system, and some of the minerals mentioned above fall into the category of electrolytes. These help transfer electrical currents between nerves and cells, affecting everything from neurologic function to muscle contractions. They are absorbed by the body with sugar and water and therefore can be easily consumed in a sports drink, whether it's a commercially available drink or one you make yourself.

There are 13 essential vitamins necessary for bodily functions. Of these, the most relevant for cyclists are vitamin B6, which helps the body's ability to transport red blood cells and oxygen to muscles; vitamin C, which is integral to building an effective immune system and aids cell repair and regeneration; vitamin D, which is useful for strengthening bones and muscles; and vitamin E, which can help to minimise the damage to cells suffered during exercise. These are all contained within the food groups that should appear in your daily meals.

Slow-release carbohydrate sources
Wholegrain breads, pasta, rice, oats, vegetables, beans, lentils, nuts.

Quick-release carbohydrate sources
Rice cakes, flapjacks, energy bars, muffins, dried fruit.

Protein sources
Eggs, fish, meat, nuts, quinoa, Greek yoghurt, cottage cheese, whey powder.

Fat sources
Nuts, seeds, avocados, olive oil, fish, meat, dairy products.

Micronutrient sources
Green leafy vegetables, legumes, nuts, seeds, other vegetables, wholegrains, fish, poultry, beef.

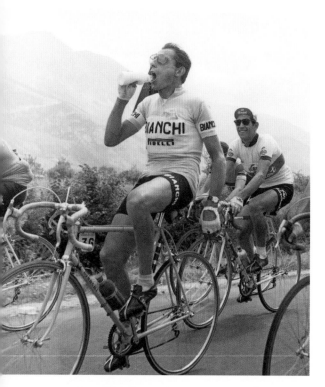

Fluid losses as small as two per cent can affect your riding performance. Refuelling on the go, Italy's cycling legend Fausto Coppi takes on water and concentrated vitamins during the 1955 Giro d'Italia. He was unable to match his triumphs of 1940, 1947, 1949, 1952 and 1953, and finished second overall.

Hydration

No matter how carefully you stick to a planned diet, it will all be for nothing if you fail to stay hydrated. I'd say that fluid losses as small as two per cent can affect your riding performance. Effective day-to-day hydration will make it easier to maintain hydration levels when you are out on the bike. Aim to take in around two to three litres of fluids a day. This will mainly be water; juices, tea, coffee and sports drinks count too, but not alcohol. Obviously, thirst indicates that you need to rehydrate, but be aware of other signs such as dryness in the mouth and less frequent trips to urinate. Check the colour of your urine: anything darker than a pale yellow is a sign you need more fluid.

If you are generally hydrated there will be no need to take on litres of water before a ride as this will only lead to 'comfort breaks' along the way. But remain alert to how much fluid you lose during a ride. You exhale moisture as you breathe, but mainly you sweat, much of which evaporates before you notice. Performance cyclists sweat sooner than non-athletes as their bodies are primed for intense exercise.

Sweat is made from blood plasma (the watery part of the blood), so replacing lost fluids will prevent the blood becoming sluggish. However, sweat also contains vital electrolytes (which give it the salty taste) and these also need replacing during a ride. Sports drinks with the correct balance of electrolytes are available or you can buy effervescent electrolyte tablets to add to your water. You can also make your own hydration drink by adding half a teaspoon of salt, two tablespoons of maple syrup and some lemon juice to half a litre of water. The contents of your bidon (water bottle) can also be used as an easy and effective way to take on extra calories or carbohydrates during a ride. Commercially available sports drinks and powders contain a mix of quick- and slower-release carbohydrates. These can be used in combination with real food, but it is important to try them in training. Different brands and ingredients suit different people and some may cause digestive distress. Find one or more you're comfortable with and stick with them.

Supplements

If you're following a balanced diet you should be able to ingest your nutritional requirements without resorting to commercial supplements. However, they can be useful as a top-up, insurance or to provide a quick energy boost.

I have mentioned carbohydrate and protein drinks, electrolyte tablets, gels and whey powder above, and they have their place during and after a ride. You might also consider nitrates, chiefly beetroot juice, which many riders find beneficial. Start loading seven days before your goal race, with two glasses of beetroot juice per day – but don't have any on race day itself, as this can cause digestive issues. Some people may also benefit from drinking a strong cup of coffee a couple of hours before a ride or a caffeine gel during a long ride, as this can not only provide mental stimulation but also stimulate the body's ability to break down fat instead of glycogen.

If you do decide to take a multivitamin supplement, choose wisely – some can contain excessively high levels of minerals that may have a negative effect on your training. A high vitamin C intake can impair training adaptation, for example, while high zinc levels can affect your body's absorption of copper and iron. Omega-3 rich fish oils might be worth considering, however, if you're not consuming much oily fish.

Some people may also benefit from drinking a strong cup of coffee a couple of hours before a ride or a caffeine gel during a long ride, as this can not only provide mental stimulation, but also stimulate the body's ability to break down fat instead of glycogen.

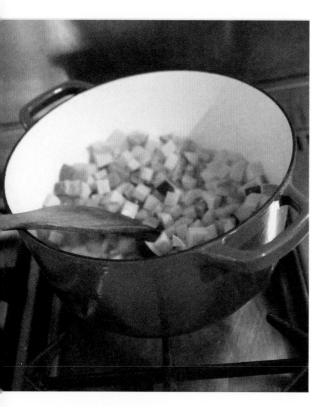

The guiding philosophy is that nutrition is not only an integral part of any athlete's planning and preparation, but also that food should satisfy the appetite and the taste buds.

What all this means for a high-performance cyclist

Calories, carbohydrates, fat, protein, vitamins, minerals, Omega-3s, fluids… it all seems like a lot of plates to keep spinning, but by following a balanced diet it can actually be relatively simple.

- Base your daily intake on a calorie ratio of 60 per cent carbohydrate, 20 per cent protein and 20 per cent fats – work on the basis that carbohydrates and protein both contain 4 calories per gram, while fats contain 9 calories per gram. Alter the ratio to suit your training and performance requirements.

- Don't obsess about losing weight. As cyclists, we need a certain amount of body fat because it is an ultra-efficient means of storing calories. A person weighing 100 kg with 10 per cent body fat has a resource of 15,000 calories to draw on.

- Stick to slow-releasing carbohydrates in your general diet and save quick-release carbs for racing or hard training days.

- Protein should be consumed regularly, but in small quantities of around 30 g per portion.

- Treat saturated fats with caution – stick to unsaturated fats as far as you can – and include as many Omega-3 foods, such as oily fish, nuts and seeds, as possible.

- Include plenty of fruit, fish, seeds and leafy vegetables to keep essential vitamin and mineral levels high.

- Maintain fluid levels at all times, but pay particular attention to rehydrating when on the bike or training.

- Include supplements only when your diet is not fulfilling nutritional requirements or when needed on the bike.

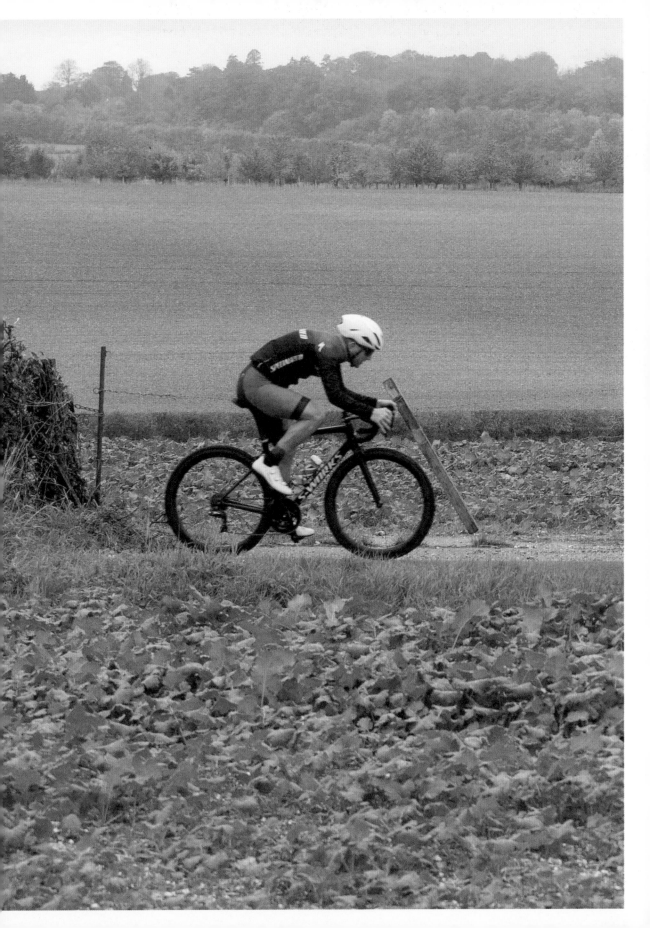

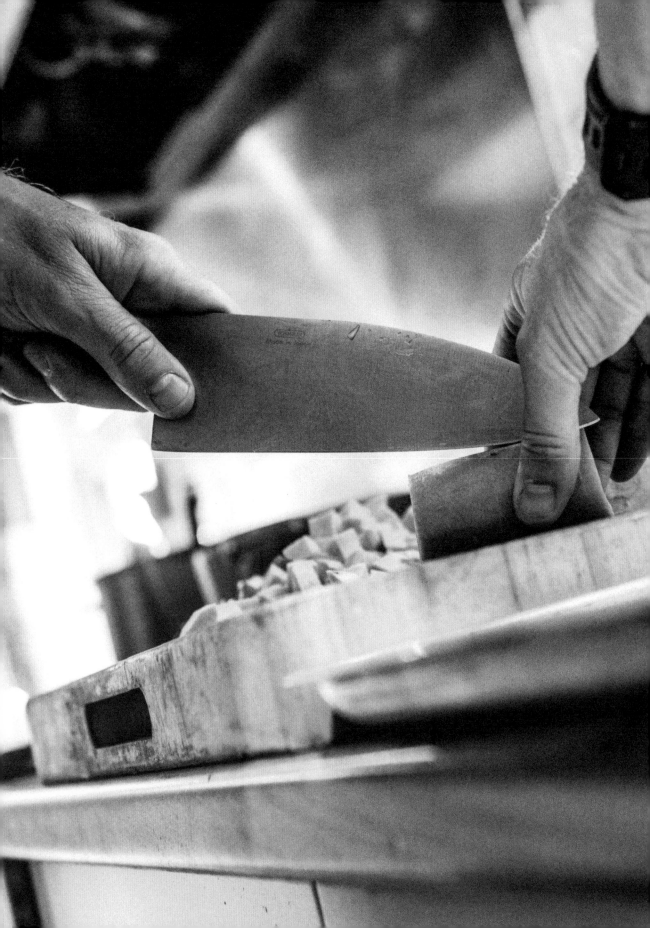

The Cyclist's Store Cupboard

It might sound like a case of 'he would say that, wouldn't he?' coming from a chef, but a fully stocked store cupboard or pantry is not a luxury but essential to any high-performance cyclist.

Fresh food is key to any high-performance diet, but a full and varied store of staples, long-life protein, spices, condiments and the odd treat will enable you to put together a meal in minutes when returning exhausted from a ride.

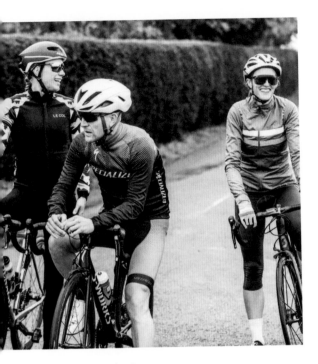

A cyclist's store cupboard should feature foodstuffs that are nutritionally rich, easy to cook and with extended sell-by dates.

Your dietary plan is demanding that every day you eat freshly cooked food containing the nutrition you require to train and perform at a high level, but we've all got better things to do than run off to the shops every mealtime. When it comes to shopping for the basics, you need to have the means at hand to cook quickly and effectively, but you also need to have a range of ingredients ready and waiting to keep your meals tasty and interesting. Fresh food – meat, fish, vegetables, fruit and dairy products – is key to any high-performance diet, but a full and varied store of staples, long-life protein, spices, condiments and the odd treat will enable you to put together a meal in minutes when returning exhausted from a ride, make a pre-ride breakfast or prepare on-the-road snacks.

A well-stocked cupboard requires foodstuffs that are nutritionally rich, easy to cook and with extended sell-by dates. Dried foods should take up plenty of shelf space, with a healthy selection of dried pasta, rice and other staples. These should mainly be wholegrain (cereal grains that include the whole kernel), which are nutrient-rich in comparison to the 'white' alternatives. Wholewheat pasta is available in all the usual shapes and sizes, brown rice comes in long-grain, jasmine and basmati forms (try red and black rice too) and you could keep wholegrain buckwheat, bulgur and couscous for variety. A small bag of white rice might come in useful if you are going to make your own rice cakes. Finally, quinoa, though technically a seed and not a grain, deserves a mention here. It is packed with more protein than any other grain and is a great source of the invaluable Omega-3 fatty acids.

Lentils are packed with nutrients, and are one of my favourite ingredients. They are rich in fibre, potassium, phosphorus, iron and copper. It's really worth getting dried lentils and taking the time to soak and cook them – the end result tastes far better than tinned lentils.

A variety of dried fruits, seeds and nuts are all handy to add to salads and bars, or to grab as a quick snack. Dried fruit carries more than 80 per cent of the nutrients of fresh fruit and is perfect in breakfasts or as a concentrated source of calories for an on-the-bike snack. Cranberries, apricots, figs and raisins are all good, or you could try the protein-rich, so-called 'superfood' goji berries. A selection of seeds will also provide a fabulous nutrient boost so keep a mix of chia seeds, flaxseed, hemp and sunflower seeds handy to grab as a quick snack or to sprinkle on your salads, porridge and smoothies. Similarly, nuts – from almond, cashew and brazil to hazelnut, pecan, pistachio and walnut – are a superb source of protein, carbs, fat, Omega-3, vitamin E and minerals. Stick to a handful a day at the most as they are high in fat and calories and eat them raw, not roasted, as they retain more nutrients and are easier to keep.

Of course, in a class of its own in terms of versatility is the humble oatmeal. Apart from being the main ingredient in bircher muesli (*see also* p. 64), oats go in homemade energy bars, smoothies, muffins and banana bread, and some riders even mix them with whey powder and milk for a post-ride recovery meal. Steel-cut and stone-ground oats are the least processed and carry the most nutrients, but beware: they can take 30 minutes or more to cook.

Moving along the shelf we find the cans. These are also your pals – you shouldn't return from any supermarket trip without a good selection of tinned beans. You can take your pick from chickpeas, kidney beans, pinto beans, soya beans, adzuki, black-eyed, haricot, butter beans – even baked beans if you have to. Packed with

A selection of seeds will also provide a fabulous nutrient boost so keep a mix of chia seeds, flaxseed, hemp and sunflower seeds handy to grab as a quick snack or to sprinkle on your salads, porridge and smoothies.

Frozen berries in particular, along with frozen whole bananas, are ideal for a quickly whipped-up smoothie and are great to have on hand in winter when fresh berries are out of season.

protein, fibre, minerals, antioxidants and slow-burning carbs, they are possibly the nearest thing you can get to a cycling superfood.

Then there's tinned fish, especially oily fish such as sardines and mackerel (although tinned tuna provides a handy protein-packed filling in a sandwich). Mash with boiled egg, serve on toast with sliced tomatoes or mix them with rice for a poor man's kedgeree. Crammed with protein, rich in Omega-3, you can't afford not to like them! If you are averse, try mixing them with some Dijon mustard and sherry vinegar.

Finally, keep a supply of tomatoes – cartons or tins. Tomatoes are an exception to the rule that cooking food reduces or destroys valuable micronutrients, as tinned tomatoes are packed with goodness. Perhaps more usefully, they are incredibly handy for a quick pasta sauce or stew.

Does the fridge count as a store cupboard? I'm going to say it does as that's where you are going to keep your eggs (just not on the inside door shelves). Eggs are a godsend. They can form a nourishing breakfast, lunch or dinner, are a fabulous convenience snack – and can be prepared and cooked in minutes. They are a complete protein package and a source of vitamins B12, D and E. However, they do vary in nutritional quality. Pastured eggs (from chickens that live outdoors for most of their lives), available from farmers' markets, as well as tasting great are richer in vitamins, but failing that, try to buy organic and beware 'free-range' – labels which can be incredibly deceptive.

Dairy products are frowned upon by some sports nutritionists, but I see no problem with moderate consumption of butter, yoghurt and milk as long as you don't have an intolerance to them. Butter, and I mean real butter, not an alternative (no matter how 'believable' it is) is rich in fat-soluble vitamins, Greek yoghurt is high in protein and is great with fruit or oats, while milk can be a good recovery drink on its own or in a smoothie. For nutritional reasons you should stick to organic milk, although soya and almond milk can provide variety as well as being a great choice for those with lactose intolerance. If you are going to opt for non-dairy milks, you will need to ensure your diet is rich in calcium from other sources. Cheese, while delicious, should be restricted to an occasional treat as it is high in fat and calories. Parmesan is perhaps the exception. Not only is it high in calcium and vitamin K and it keeps for ages, but it's also culinary magic – just a small amount can make most meals appetising! Meanwhile, if you have freezer space, it can be usefully filled with bags of peas and sweetcorn and frozen fruit, which contains barely fewer nutrients than fresh fruit. Frozen berries in particular, along with frozen whole bananas, are ideal for a quickly whipped-up smoothie and are great to have on hand in winter when fresh berries are out of season.

The key to being able to prepare a good meal with all the above is the oils, condiments, herbs and spices that bring out the flavour in food. Use regular olive oil for cooking, save good-quality virgin olive oil for using cold. Don't bother with dried herbs – the flavour isn't good enough to serve any real purpose – and stick to good-quality stock cubes for soups and stews. If you can, buy Himalayan salt, the most unprocessed salt you can get, and use honey (preferably Manuka honey, though it is expensive) or maple syrup as an alternative to sugar. Other items are down to personal taste – mustards, soy sauce and vinegars can all pep up an otherwise bland meal. Have some fun working your way through the supermarket spice selection and discover some favourite seasonings. Look especially for turmeric, whose active component curcumin is great for helping to soothe post-cycle inflammation, and cinnamon,

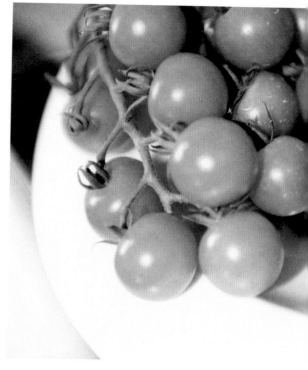

Tomatoes – fresh or tinned – are packed with goodness and they are incredibly handy for a quick pasta sauce or stew.

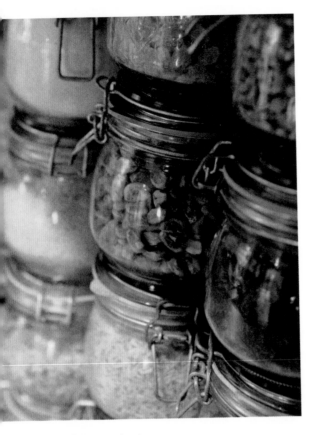

In a cyclist's store cupboard, dried foods should take up plenty of shelf space, with a healthy selection of pasta, rice and other staples. A range of seeds and nuts will also provide a fabulous nutrient boost.

which can help your body to regulate its blood glucose levels.

Finally, remember to keep a good supply of snacks and on-the-bike supplies (*see also* p. 154) – not only nut butter, fig roll biscuits and rice cakes, but also any specialist products such as electrolyte tablets, protein powder, energy bars and gels you might need.

Store Cupboard Essentials

Dried goods: Brown rice, wholemeal pasta, quinoa, amaranth (a type of grain), buckwheat noodles, red and green lentils.

Canned beans: Baked beans, chickpeas, kidney beans, adzuki, cannellini and any other bean that looks interesting.

Canned fish: Mackerel, tuna, anchovies, sardines (if you can't handle the taste, mix with a touch of Dijon mustard, sherry vinegar and olive oil).

Dried fruit: Dates, figs, raisins, apricots, cranberries, bananas, blueberries, goji berries.

Nuts and seeds: Cashews, walnuts, hazelnuts, almonds, flaxseed, sesame, pumpkin, hemp and chia seeds.

Fridge: Butter, Greek yoghurt, organic milk, almond milk, Parmesan, eggs, fresh pesto.

Freezer: Peas, sweetcorn, fruit, mixed berries, whole bananas.

Sundries: Olive oil (normal and extra virgin), stock cubes, Manuka honey, maple syrup, Dijon mustard, sherry vinegar, Himalayan salt, peanut butter, Marmite, spices.

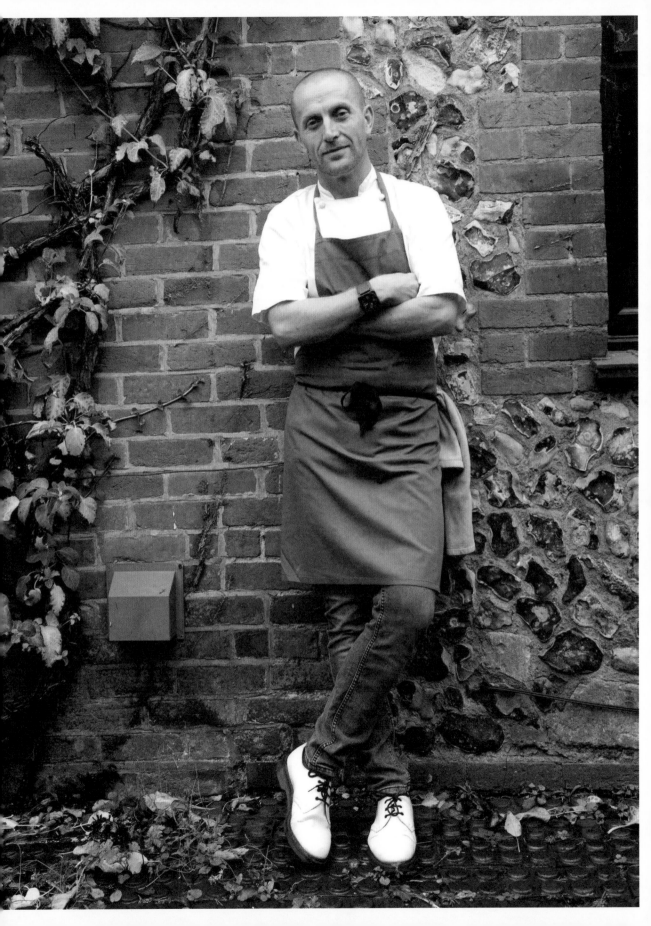

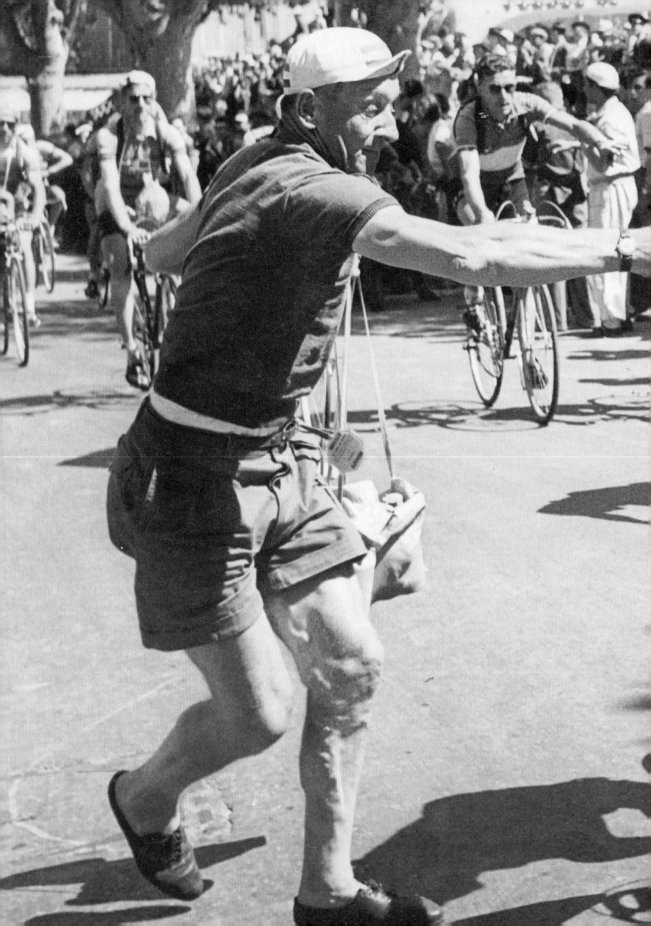

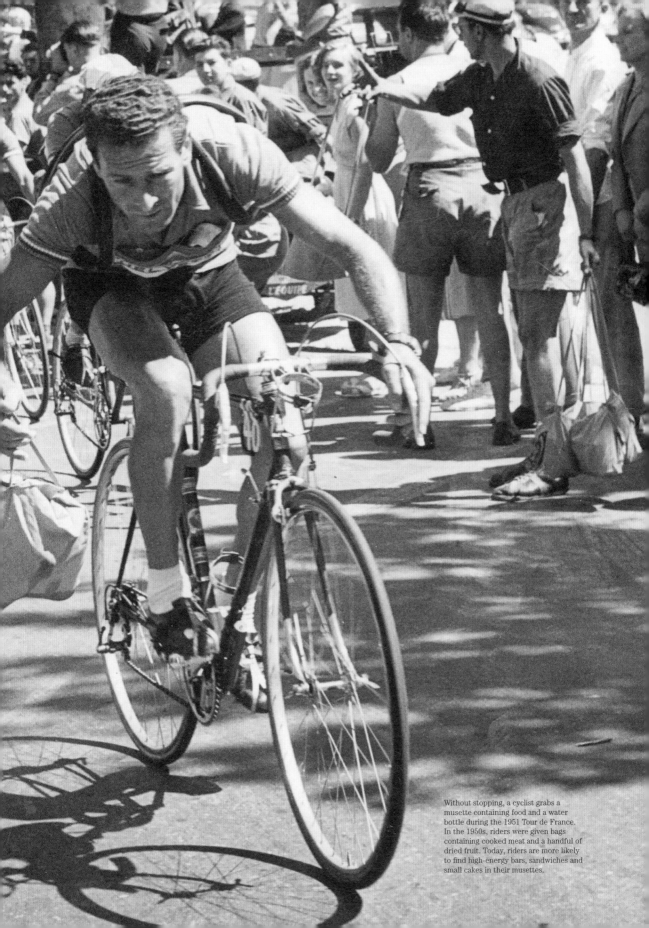

Without stopping, a cyclist grabs a musette containing food and a water bottle during the 1951 Tour de France. In the 1950s, riders were given bags containing cooked meat and a handful of dried fruit. Today, riders are more likely to find high-energy bars, sandwiches and small cakes in their musettes.

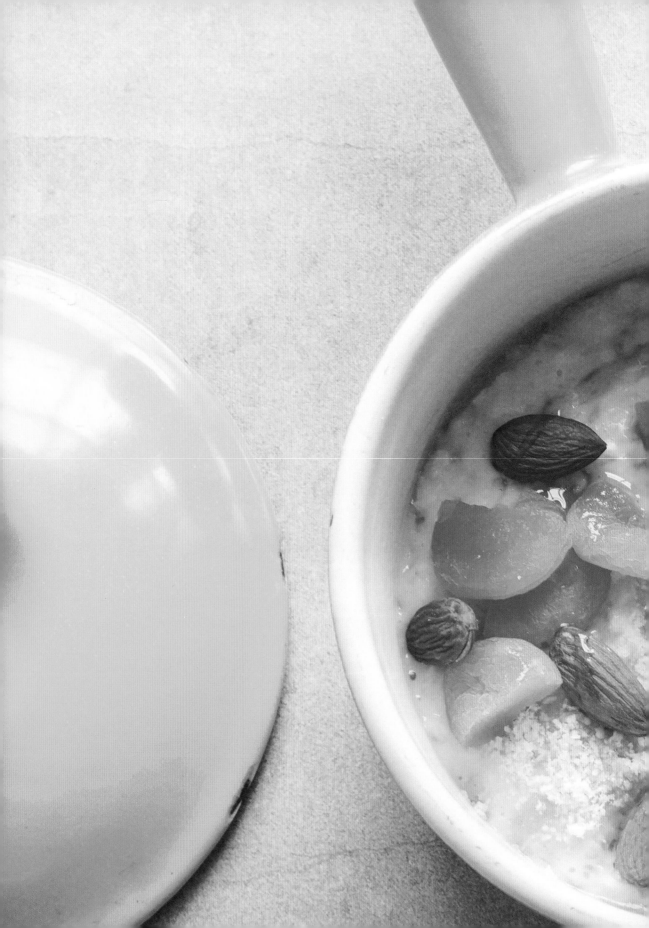

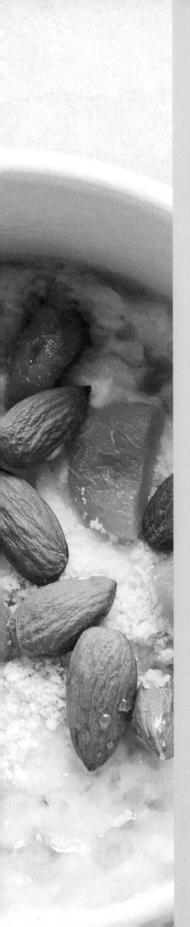

Breakfasts

The options for the first meal of the day are varied and delicious – from oats to eggs to toast and smoothies – and breakfast is a perfect opportunity to consume some essential nutrients.

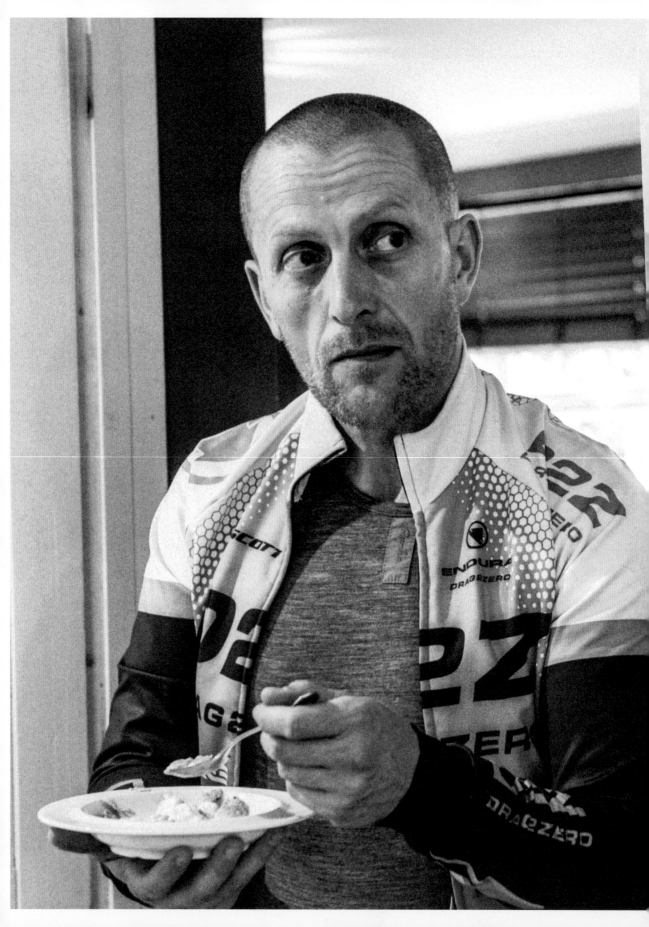

As cyclist nutritional rules go, this one is basic: you can't afford to skip breakfast. You've just gone half a day without sustenance, while your body burns 50 to 100 calories an hour and uses protein resources to repair your muscles while you sleep. You've got to eat something!

Most nutritionists agree that we should aim to consume around 20 per cent of our daily energy intake at breakfast. This provides a key opportunity to take in the balance of nutrients we need, so any breakfast should ideally include a slow-release carbohydrate, protein and fruit.

Like all meals, breakfast should reflect your training. A light breakfast will suffice for rest days, with a more hearty meal necessary at least 90 minutes before setting off for a training ride or club session. Race day might require a more substantial breakfast two to three hours before the start. This should be based on slow-release carbohydrates, but also include protein and fruit.

What you eat is largely down to personal choice. Many of us find it difficult to think further than cereal, eggs or toast, but we can easily work with that (let's keep a fry-up for an occasional treat). Oatmeal is God's gift to cyclists. Eggs are protein rich, while wholemeal toast can provide a great nutritional base. Around the world, however, breakfasts might include cold meats, rice, vegetables or soup – so why not broaden your cultural boundaries.

Breakfast can be a rushed affair. But you can prepare something quickly or have a pre-cooked snack that can be eaten on the move. Bircher muesli can sit in the fridge overnight, or you can easily whizz up an energising smoothie.

Enjoying your breakfast is essential. Skip breakfast and you will have difficulty satisfying your body's nutritional demands for the day, so make sure you have a wide range of easily prepared fresh foods to choose from.

Like all meals, breakfast should reflect your training. A light breakfast will suffice for rest days, with a more hearty meal necessary at least 90 minutes before setting off for a training ride.

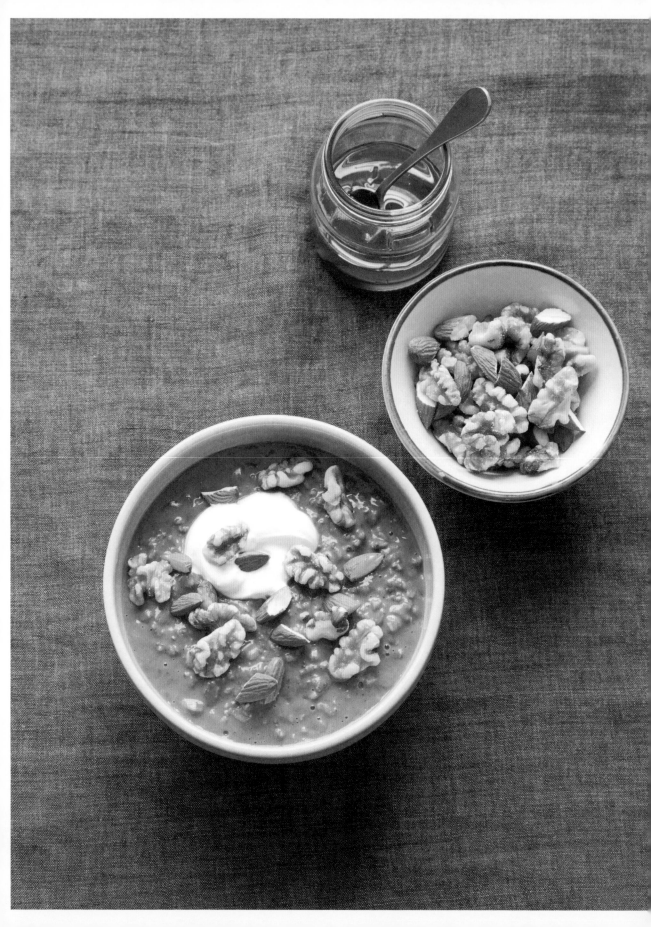

Power porridge with chocolate, chia seeds and almond butter

A filling and rich breakfast – the perfect start to the day ahead and a long ride on the bike

Chocolate milk and almond butter are an excellent pairing, and the addition of chopped banana would also work really well. Manuka honey is loaded with antioxidants to boost your energy levels.

Serves 1

65 g (2 ½ oz) oats

120 ml (½ cup) water

200 ml (¾ cup) chocolate soya milk

1 teaspoon cocoa nibs (Grue de Cacao)

1 tablespoon almond butter

2 teaspoons chia seeds

1 tablespoon low-fat Greek yoghurt

1 teaspoon Manuka honey

2 tablespoons mixed nuts (almonds and walnuts are ideal)

1. Place the oats, water, chocolate soya milk and cocoa nibs in a medium saucepan. Cook over a low heat for 10 minutes, stirring occasionally. Add a touch more water if required.

2. When cooked, stir in the almond butter and chia seeds.

3. Serve with the Greek yoghurt, Manuka honey and nuts.

Nutrition per serving:

Calories 712 | Total carbohydrate 75 g | Sugars 25 g
Fat 33 g | Protein 28 g | Sodium 0 mg

Multiseed pancakes

Great for a pre-ride quality breakfast or as a post-ride lunch

Making a good pancake is a great skill to master and this recipe could not be easier. You can make the mix up in advance, cover and store in the fridge overnight. Then, freestyle with the toppings – banana, Greek yoghurt and maple syrup; fresh fruit, honey and crème fraîche – or you could go savoury with smoked salmon, chopped dill, capers and natural yoghurt.

**Makes 6 x 125 g (4 oz) pancakes
(2 pancakes = a normal breakfast,
3 = full-on!)**

4 large free-range eggs

250 ml (1 cup) milk (can be substituted with a non-dairy milk; unsweetened almond milk works particularly well)

230 g (8 oz) gluten-free
self-raising flour

1 teaspoon chia seeds

1 teaspoon hemp seeds

1 teaspoon pumpkin seeds

1 teaspoon sunflower seeds

1 tablespoon olive oil

Nutrition per serving (2 pancakes):
Calories 478 | Total carbohydrate 68 g | Sugars 4 g
Fat 16 g | Protein 16 g | Sodium 181 mg

1. Crack the eggs into a large mixing bowl, then whisk in the milk.

2. Gradually incorporate the flour until you have a smooth paste.

3. Add the mixed seeds and allow to sit for 5 minutes.

4. Preheat a medium non-stick sauté pan. Add a little oil to form a very light coating on the base of the pan. Pour out any excess oil and reserve for the next pancake (you really only need a very small amount).

5. Ladle in 125 ml (½ cup) of the pancake mix (basically, 1 medium ladle) and fry for 2 minutes on each side until golden brown. Stack between sheets of greaseproof paper on a plate fitted over a pan of simmering water to keep warm while you make the rest.

6. Serve with your favourite toppings. These pancakes are great to make in advance and freeze – just stack them between sheets of greaseproof paper and put them in an airtight container or freezer bag, and you'll have an easy-to-grab meal.

Mango, pineapple and passion fruit grain porridge

This tropical porridge-type dish is a great pre-race or mid-afternoon filler

Easily digestible, with a lovely texture, if you are looking for a richer flavour, replace the Greek yoghurt with creamed coconut. White chia seeds give a hearty dose of Omega-3, fibre and protein.

Serves 1

65 g (2 ½ oz) quick-cook corn, bulgur and red quinoa mix

1 teaspoon flax seeds

1 teaspoon white chia seeds

150 ml (½ cup) pineapple juice

150 ml (½ cup) mango and apple juice

50 ml (3 tablespoons) water

1 tablespoon low-fat Greek yoghurt

50 g (2 oz) fresh chopped pineapple

50 g (2 oz) fresh chopped mango

Seeds and flesh of 1 large passion fruit

12 cashew nuts, whole

1 teaspoon desiccated coconut

1. Place the corn, bulgur and red quinoa mix, flax seeds, white chia seeds, fruit juices and water in a saucepan. Simmer for 12–15 minutes, stirring occasionally, until the grains are cooked and the liquid has been absorbed.

2. Allow to cool for 5 minutes, then stir in the Greek yoghurt.

3. Finish by pouring into a bowl and top with the fresh fruit, cashews and coconut to serve.

Nutrition per serving:

Calories 528 | Total carbohydrate 84 g | Sugars 47 g
Fat 13 g | Protein 14 g | Sodium 190 mg

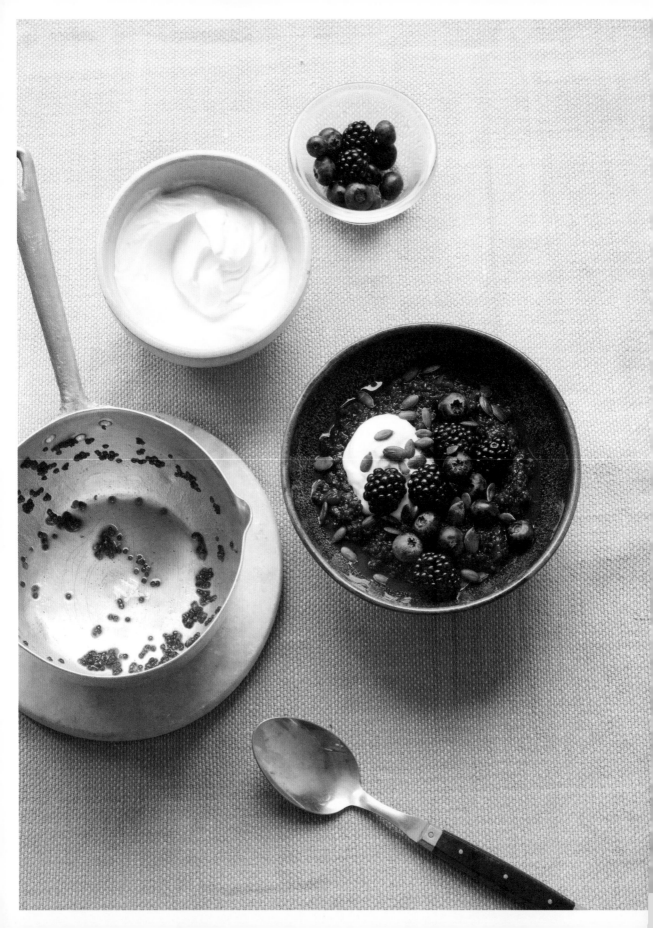

Beetroot and cherry porridge

As well as being a vibrant start to the day, this 'porridge' works really well as a mid-afternoon snack ahead of a hard session

Please don't turn the page when you see the words 'beetroot' and 'porridge' in the same line. As all of us cyclist types know, porridge is a staple of any balanced diet. Beetroot is really good for you and helps balance out the sweetness of the apple juice. It's also one of your daily veg. As the porridge takes about 20 minutes to cook, it can be made up in advance and eats really well cold.

Serves 1

65 g (2 ½ oz) red quinoa

30 g (1 oz) dried cherries

1 teaspoon chia seeds

1 teaspoon concentrated beetroot juice

250 ml (1 cup) apple juice

100 ml (½ cup) water

1 heaped tablespoon Greek yoghurt

1 teaspoon pumpkin seeds

75 g (3 oz) fresh blueberries and blackberries

1. Mix together the red quinoa, dried cherries, chia seeds, concentrated beetroot juice, apple juice and water in a saucepan. Simmer gently for 16–18 minutes.

2. Allow to sit for 5 minutes, for the quinoa to absorb the liquid. Once the quinoa is tender, pour into a bowl. Spoon over the yoghurt and top with pumpkin seeds and fresh berries to serve.

Nutrition per serving:
Calories 569 | Total carbohydrate 116 g | Sugars 58 g
Fat 9 g | Protein 15 g | Sodium 4 mg

Rice flake, almond and apricot porridge

Easy-to-cook rice flakes are a welcome alternative to oats for a delicious kickstart to the day

Any time we can create a breakfast dessert, we are truly on to a winner! This is almost like having rice pudding for breakfast. The recipe is also gluten-free and vegan. For a slightly sweeter taste, add a touch more maple syrup before serving.

Serves 1

60 g (2 ½ oz) rice flakes

210 ml (¾ cup) almond milk

1 tablespoon maple syrup

1 teaspoon flax seeds

1 tablespoon ground almonds

15 g (½ oz) whole almonds

40 g (1 ½ oz) dried apricots

Nutrition per serving:
Calories 653 | Total carbohydrate 88 g | Sugars 32 g
Fat 22 g | Protein 16 g | Sodium 128 mg

1. Place the rice flakes, almond milk, maple syrup and flax seeds in a medium saucepan. Cook over a low to medium heat for 8–10 minutes, stirring occasionally.

2. Pour the porridge into a bowl and serve sprinkled with ground and whole almonds and apricots.

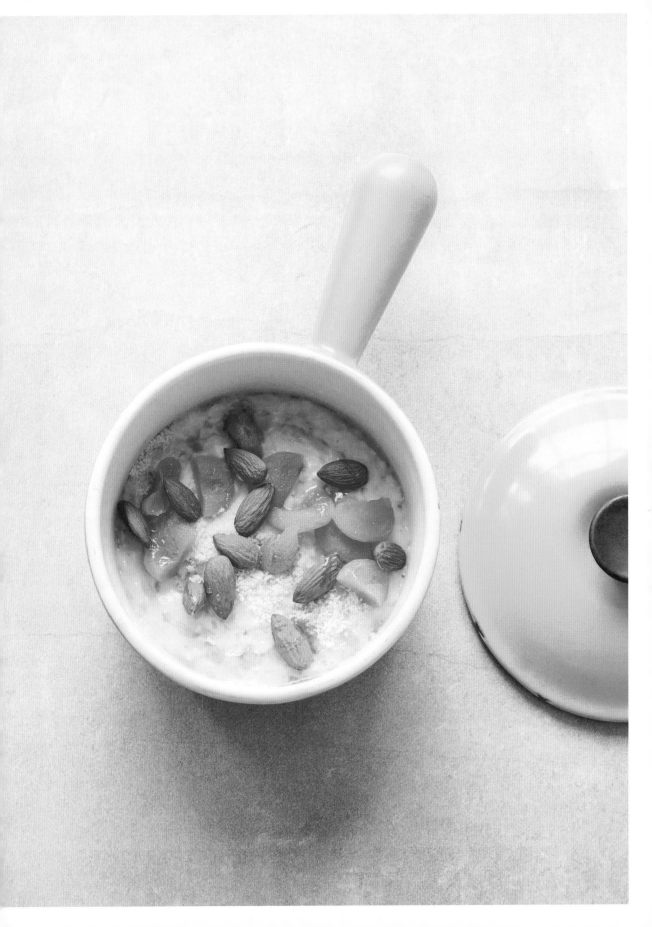

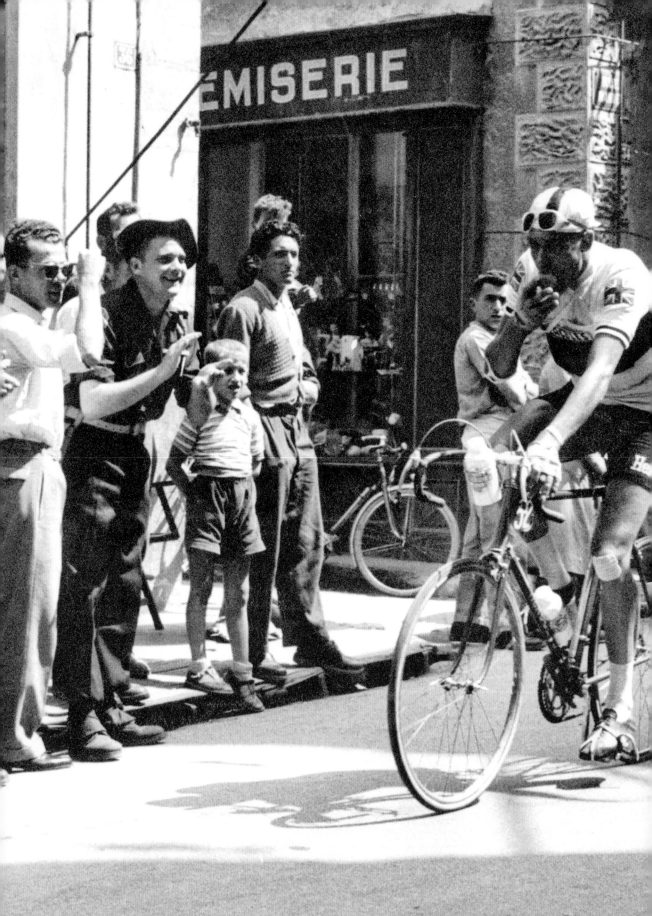

Special Diets and the Elite Athlete

The exclusion of any food group presents a challenge for a high-performance athlete, so how do ethical and medical exclusions affect performance and recovery?

Can you be a high-performance athlete and exclude certain foods from your diet? The short answer is, yes, you can. There are examples of vegetarians, vegans and competitors with other exclusive diets among elite endurance sports – but they are few and far between. In my five years advising Olympians and professional athletes, I can count the number of vegetarians and vegans I have worked with on one hand. And there's a good reason: it's a near-impossible challenge. I know – I've tried training and competing without meat and dairy myself and the truth is it's bloody difficult!

British rider Tony Hoar sucks a tomato on his way through a southern French village during the 1955 Tour de France. Adopting a vegan or vegetarian diet is challenging for high-performance athletes and may leave them at a disadvantage.

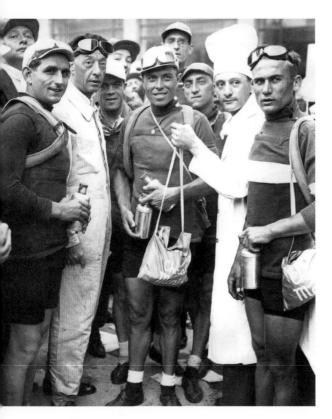

Italian cyclist Learco Guerra poses in the yellow jersey with his musette in 1930. An elite cyclist has to make many compromises in terms of financial, social and even career choices, and, unfortunately, dietary ethics may be just one more sacrifice that has to be added to that list.

I totally understand the ethical and moral arguments associated with meat- and dairy-free diets, but I also believe that to maintain a high-performance diet you cannot exclude essential foods. Meat, fish and eggs come pretty high up that list. Eighty per cent of my store cupboard might be vegan, but any diet plan I produce for an elite cyclist will be fully balanced – and that means red and white meat and fish.

Red meat, in particular, is rich in iron, an important component of haemoglobin, the protein in red blood cells that transports oxygen around the body. Iron from plant or dairy sources, or from supplements, is much less easily absorbed into the bloodstream. Zinc, again most commonly found in meats, can act as both an antioxidant and anti-inflammatory, while vitamin B12, which cannot be obtained from any plant food, is necessary for energy production. Finally, meats alone contain creatine, which helps muscles produce energy during high-intensity exercise – important for any athlete.

A carefully constructed diet, and the use of various supplements, may be able to match the benefits of a diet featuring meat. But you need to be pretty dedicated to attempt this. An elite cyclist has to make many compromises in terms of financial, social and even career choices, and unfortunately, I consider dietary ethics as just one more sacrifice that has to be added to that list.

However, it is important to look after your gut. When you consider that strenuous exercise directs blood flow away from the digestive system to the muscles, it's unsurprising that some riders suffer from digestive problems. The gut is key to the fuelling of the body and anything you can do to maintain its condition can help improve your performance on the bike.

Bread and pasta, many athletes' major source of carbohydrates, contain wheat gluten – the protein that makes baked goods light and chewy – which some people find difficult to digest. Could a gluten-free diet improve performance? Some people believe it eases digestion and enhances the body's absorption of nutrients. Indeed, going gluten-free has become a trend among endurance athletes around the world, including several pro-cycling teams. I was sceptical, so I tried it (just to prove it wouldn't work) but after a few weeks I have to admit it definitely improved my digestion.

Before excluding any food from your diet, you should always seek advice from a registered nutritionist, dietician or doctor. If you select healthy alternatives, a gluten-free diet can be undertaken without excluding any vital nutrients, but it needs to be done carefully to ensure you don't miss out on anything important. Breads, pasta, crackers and cereals are easily substituted with rice, potatoes, tortillas and gluten-free breads and pasta (although remember to check the nutrition stats of any processed products). You will also need to maintain your fibre intake with vegetables and fruit. It may not work for everyone, but there is no harm in giving it a go for a few weeks as long as you plan accordingly.

A similar argument could be made for trying a lactose-free (non-dairy) diet as it's also a possible source of digestive distress. However, dairy products have a significant impact on energy, carbohydrate and protein values and contribute significantly to recovery. Non-dairy sources of calcium can be found in canned fish, dried fruit or leafy vegetables, and other nutrients may be boosted by supplements, but this is not ideal in a high-performance diet. By all means cut down on dairy by alternating cow's milk with alternatives such as soya, brown rice or almond milk (ensure these are fortified with calcium) but, unless it is a medical issue, don't erase it from your diet completely.

Food Exclusion Rules

- Don't exclude meat, fish or dairy from your diet unless it is medically or ethically impossible to avoid doing so.
- Consider reducing your intake of certain food groups instead of eliminating them from your diet.
- Understand which nutrients you're missing and how you'll compensate.
- Ensure you're not over-consuming carbohydrates, fat or sugars to compensate for missing nutrients.
- Check the protein content of replacement foodstuffs.
- Avoid highly processed meat-, dairy- or gluten-free alternatives.

Vegetarian Essentials

The following foods should be regularly consumed by any athlete undertaking a vegetarian diet:

- Eggs
- Dairy
- Pulses
- Nuts and seeds
- Quinoa and buckwheat
- Spinach, broccoli and kale
- Soya products – for example tofu and soya milk.

Gluten-free Alternatives

- Rice
- Potatoes
- Sweet potatoes
- Gluten-free breads and pasta
- Quinoa and buckwheat
- Polenta
- Porridge oats.

Vegan banana pancakes

The banana is a nutritional powerhouse, packed with energy-giving carbs and an excellent source of potassium too

These pancakes have a very different texture to regular ones, being slightly denser. They are also great if you stir some dried fruit into the mix. They are best made and eaten immediately, as the texture becomes rubbery if left to cool.

Makes 3–4 medium pancakes

225 g (8 oz) gluten-free self-raising flour

225 ml (¾ cup) soya milk

a pinch of sea salt

2 tablespoons dried coconut

1 large ripe banana, peeled

1 tablespoon melted coconut oil

1 teaspoon olive oil (extra for frying)

Fresh fruit to serve (such as one sliced banana or 50 g / 2 oz of seasonal berries)

Nutrition per serving (1 pancake):

Calories 339 | Total carbohydrate 56 g | Sugars 7 g
Fat 11 g | Protein 5 g | Sodium 330 mg

1. In a food processor, whizz all ingredients to form a smooth paste.

2. Preheat a medium non-stick sauté pan. Add a small splash of olive oil to form a light coating on the base of the pan. Pour away any excess oil, reserving it for the next pancake (you really only need a very small amount).

3. Ladle in 125 ml (½ cup) of the mix (basically, 1 medium ladle). Fry for 2 minutes on each side until golden brown.

4. Serve at once with fresh fruit.

Cinnamon and sesame French toast

An awesome breakfast ahead of a big day in the saddle!

This is a great way of using up bread that is not quite as fresh as it could be. You can easily make a savoury French toast and serve with grilled tomatoes and sautéed button mushrooms – obviously leave out the cinnamon, nutmeg and sugar!

Serves 2

3 eggs, beaten

2 tablespoons milk

1 teaspoon ground cinnamon

a pinch of ground nutmeg

1 tablespoon sesame seeds

1 tablespoon brown sugar

4 thick slices hand-cut, good-quality bread (ideally 2 days old)

1 teaspoon olive oil

Greek yoghurt and/or a good-quality maple syrup or honey to serve

Nutrition per serving:
Calories 399 | Total carbohydrate 49 g | Sugars 9 g
Fat 15 g | Protein 19 g | Sodium 109 mg

1. Whisk together in a large bowl the eggs, milk, cinnamon, nutmeg, sesame seeds and brown sugar.

2. Dip the slices of bread in the egg mixture, ensuring they are well-coated and the egg mix has soaked in.

3. Preheat a large non-stick sauté pan. Add the olive oil to form a very light coating on the base of the pan. Pour out any excess oil and reserve for the next slice (you only need a very small amount).

4. Fry each slice of soaked bread over a medium heat for 2–3 minutes on each side until golden.

5. Serve topped with Greek yoghurt and/or maple syrup or honey.

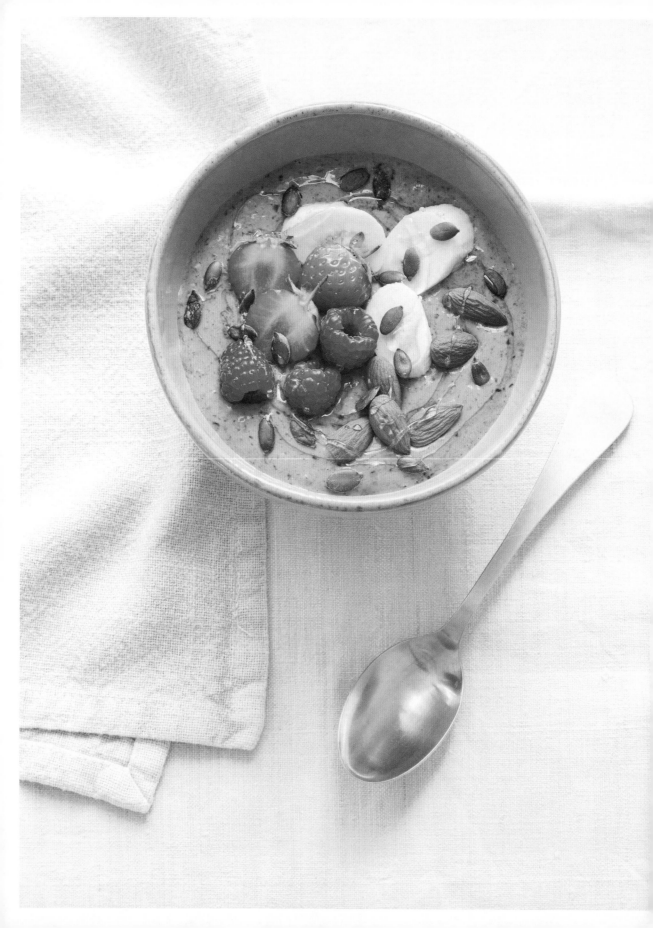

Smoothie bowl

Frozen berries pack as much of a nutritional punch as fresh berries, without the risk of them spoiling before you have a chance to use them all up

A more robust version of a smoothie, think of this as a wet-fruit muesli! It's an excellent way of using up leftover fruit, but I always like to keep a selection of frozen fruit in stock. Blueberries, raspberries and mixed summer fruits are great go-tos and must-have items in any busy cyclist's freezer.

Serves 1

50 ml (3 tablespoons) almond milk

100 g (3 ½ oz) frozen berries such as blueberries or raspberries (or most supermarkets stock a 'smoothie mix' of mixed fruits)

1 banana, peeled

a handful of spinach leaves

1 tablespoon rolled oats

20 g (¾ oz) chia seeds

100 g (3 ½ oz) low-fat Greek yoghurt

1 tablespoon mixed seeds such as sunflower or pumpkin seeds

fresh berries (halved strawberries, whole raspberries), banana slices, pumpkin seeds, almonds (whole, skin on), and honey, as liked, to serve

1. In a food processor, blend together the almond milk, frozen berries, banana and spinach leaves.

2. Stir in the oats, chia seeds, Greek yoghurt and mixed seeds. Transfer to a bowl and leave to set in the fridge for 30 minutes.

3. Serve with fresh berries, banana slices, pumpkin seeds, almonds and honey to taste.

Nutrition per serving:
Calories 399 | Total carbohydrate 56 g | Sugars 24 g
Fat 11 g | Protein 21 g | Sodium 56 mg

Kedgeree

My take on a classic Scottish dish (yes, it is Scottish originally), this is perfect training food as it's a great mix of slow-release carbs with loads of protein

Traditionally, kedgeree uses basmati rice, a much more delicate grain than Arborio (risotto) or long-grain rice – take care when stirring and cooking as it will easily break up. From start to finish, this dish takes less than 20 minutes to cook.

Serves 2 (with a portion left for lunch)

25 g (1 oz) butter

1 onion, peeled and finely chopped

2 teaspoons medium curry powder (nothing too spicy or abrasive)

1 teaspoon ground turmeric

200 g (7 oz) basmati rice

600 ml (2 ½ cups) fish or vegetable stock (good-quality stock cubes or shop-bought stock)

400 g (14 oz) smoked haddock fillet, skin removed (you can ask your fishmonger to do this), trimmed and diced

200 g (7 oz) frozen peas

1 bunch of spring onions, trimmed and chopped

3–4 large free-range eggs, soft-boiled and halved

1 teaspoon black onion seeds

1 tablespoon sultanas

Nutrition per serving:
Calories 592 | Total carbohydrate 71 g | Sugars 8 g
Fat 16 g | Protein 43 g | Sodium 1486 mg

1. Preheat a large non-stick pan and melt the butter over a low heat. Fry the onion until softened, about 2–3 minutes. Stir in the curry powder and turmeric; cook for a further 2 minutes.

2. Now add the rice and stir well. Pour in the stock and simmer for 10 minutes, stirring occasionally. When the rice is 85 per cent there (basmati usually cooks for 12 minutes, follow the instructions on the packet), add the smoked haddock and peas. Stir in very gently and reduce the heat to low. Simmer for 2–3 minutes to cook the haddock (it will go from being opaque to white – take care not to overcook it).

3. Just before serving, stir in the chopped spring onions and serve topped with boiled egg halves and a sprinkling of onion seeds and sultanas.

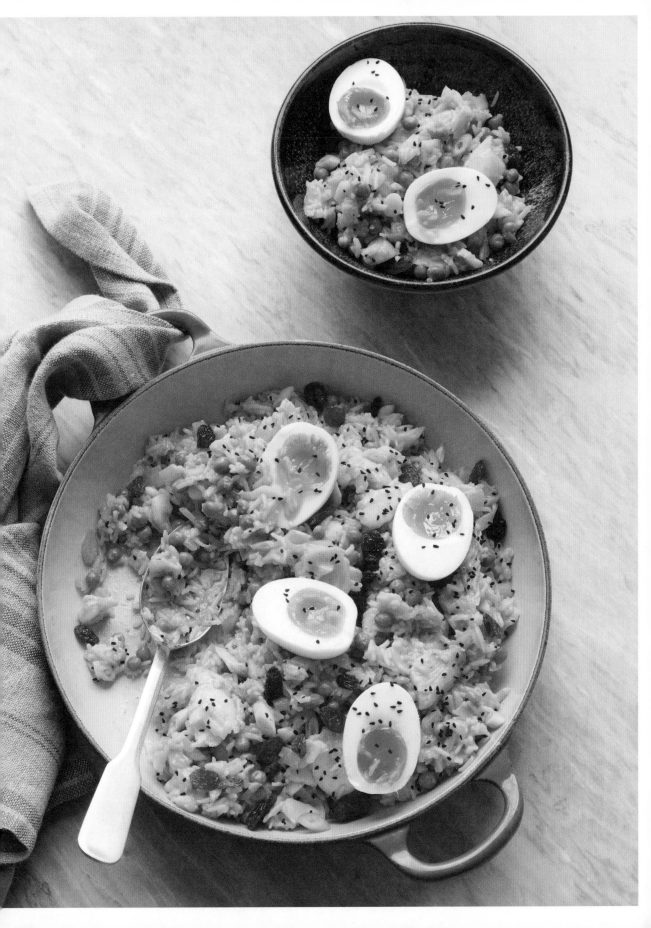

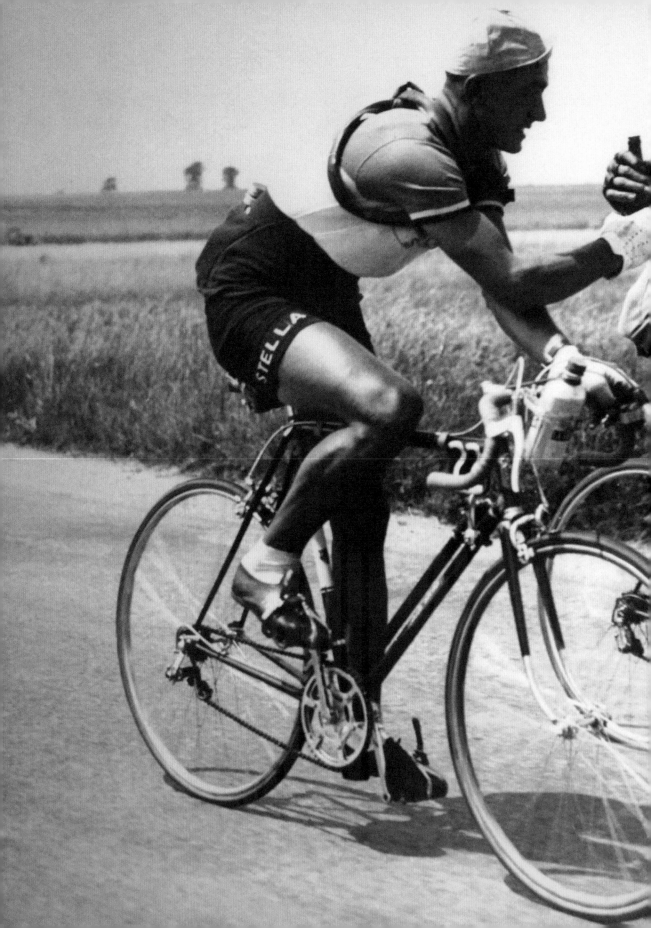

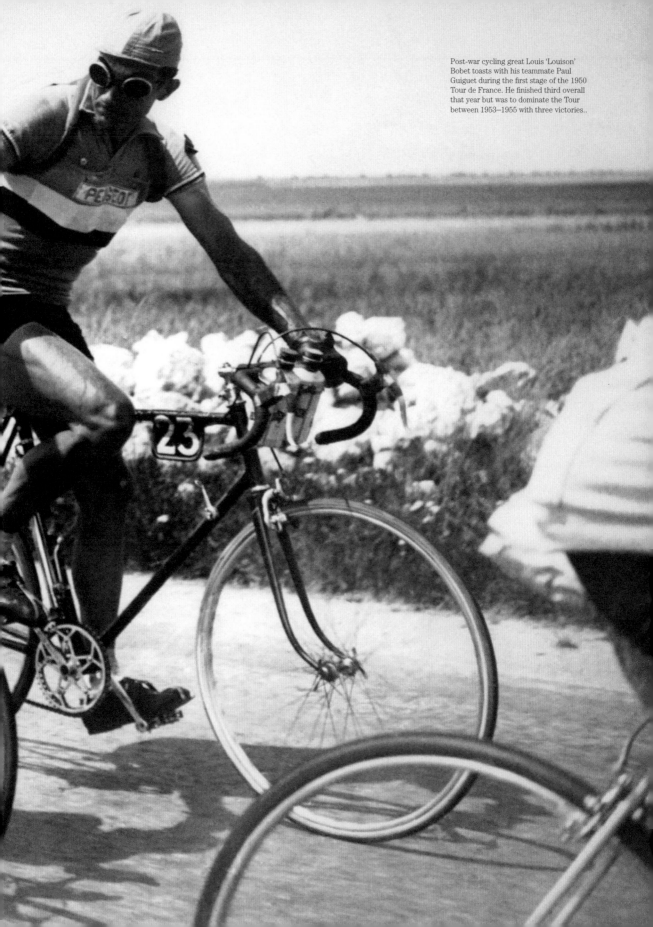

Post-war cycling great Louis 'Louison' Bobet toasts with his teammate Paul Guiguet during the first stage of the 1950 Tour de France. He finished third overall that year but was to dominate the Tour between 1953–1955 with three victories..

Bircher muesli

For me, bircher muesli is one of the best ways to start the day. It can be made in advance and uses simple ingredients that can be found anywhere. It's a great mix of slow- and quick-release carbs, fat, protein – and also very tasty. Bircher was invented by the Swiss physician Maximilian Bircher-Benner around 1900. He believed raw foods are more nutritious as they contain direct energy from the sun. Max was actually way ahead of his time with regard to the raw food movement; one of the original hipsters!

After lots of experimentation I have found that bircher is easy to digest and sits really well in the stomach when cycling. It tends to leave me feeling less bloated than porridge, for example. It also works really well for an afternoon snack if you have an evening race, or when you're just having one of those hungry days. Bircher is often eaten in the evenings in Europe.

A really simple base is 50 g (2 oz) oats, 50 g (2 oz) yoghurt and 100 ml (½ cup) of milk or fruit juice. This will give you a good start when it comes to adding your own flavour and texture combinations. You can easily increase the protein levels by adding chia or hemp seeds. If you need a slightly more filling breakfast, add some ground almonds or coconut flakes. Have a play and see what you come up with.

The process for each of these recipes is the same: mix all the ingredients together, cover and place in the fridge overnight. Alternatively, you can make it up in the morning and leave for 15–20 minutes. If leaving overnight, you might need to add a splash (25 ml / 1 ½ tablespoons) of milk in the morning as the oats soak up a lot of liquid when left. I prefer to add nuts at the last minute as I like the crunchy texture.

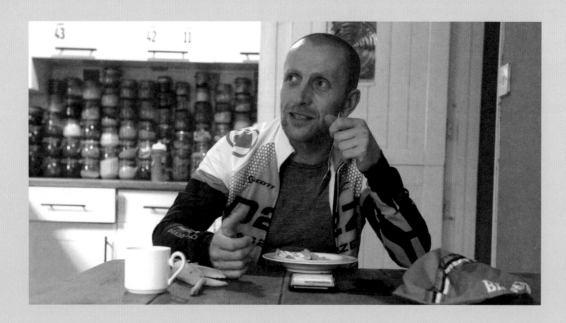

Mocha bircher

Perfect for pumping adrenalin levels, you can never have too much coffee in your life!

Chocolate for breakfast… living the dream! Add a teaspoon of Grue de Cacao (cocoa nibs) if you want some more texture and a really deep bitter chocolate flavour.

Serves 1

60 g (2 ½ oz) gluten-free oats

2 teaspoons ground almonds

1 tablespoon chia seeds

2 teaspoons 'Sweet Freedom' vegan hot chocolate shot

60 g (2 ½ oz) soya yoghurt

1 shot espresso coffee (or 1 tablespoon strong instant coffee)

100 ml (½ cup) chocolate soya milk

a handful of walnuts, hazelnuts and almonds, to serve

Nutrition per serving:
Calories 555 | Total carbohydrate 55 g | Sugars 15 g
Fat 27 g | Protein 22 g | Sodium 61 mg

1. Weigh out your dry ingredients – oats, ground almonds and chia seeds – into your breakfast bowl.

2. Stir in the wet ingredients.

3. Leave to sit for 10 minutes at room temperature or overnight in the fridge. If leaving overnight in the fridge you may need to add an extra splash of milk in the morning. The texture should resemble a loose porridge.

4. Top with the nuts just before eating to make sure the nuts retain their crunch.

Piña colada bircher

This bircher could also be a great pre-bed dessert ahead of a heavy day on the bike

It feels like a treat for breakfast, but tropical fruit is available all year round and relatively cheap to buy. This recipe also works well with mango and apple juice or even full-on canned coconut milk, which will increase the calorie count considerably. However, that could be a good thing ahead of a long ride. For added texture, stir in a few cashew nuts just before serving.

Serves 1

50 g (2 oz) gluten-free oats

1 tablespoon chia seeds

1 tablespoon desiccated coconut

50 g (2 oz) low-fat Greek yoghurt

50 ml (3 tablespoons) coconut soya milk (or brown rice milk)

50 ml (3 tablespoons) pineapple juice

1 banana, peeled and sliced

150 g (5 oz) chopped fresh pineapple and mango

1. Weigh out the oats, chia seeds and desiccated coconut into your breakfast bowl.

2. Stir in the wet ingredients and sliced banana.

3. Leave to sit for 10 minutes at room temperature or overnight in the fridge. If leaving overnight in the fridge you may need to add an extra splash of milk in the morning. The texture should resemble a loose porridge.

4. Top with fresh pineapple and mango to serve.

Nutrition per serving:
Calories 659 | Total carbohydrate 100 g | Sugars 44 g
Fat 21 g | Protein 20 g | Sodium 53 mg

Classic apple and cinnamon bircher

We use this as a pre-race breakfast – it goes down really easy, with no strong flavours to worry about

Really simple, classic flavours and easy to throw together, but if you want to try something different, replace the milk with apple juice. Serve with a tablespoon of flaked almonds and a teaspoon of honey if you prefer a slightly sweeter breakfast.

Serves 1

50 g (2 oz) gluten-free oats

25 g (1 oz) raisins

a pinch of cinnamon

1 large apple, skin on, grated

100 ml (½ cup) semi-skimmed milk (can be substituted with a non-dairy milk; unsweetened almond milk works particularly well)

50 g (2 oz) Greek yoghurt

1. Weigh out your dry ingredients – oats, raisins and cinnamon – into your breakfast bowl.

2. Grate your apple into the bowl. Leaving the skin on gives a really nice texture and also retains more nutrients.

3. Add the milk and yoghurt.

4. Leave to sit for 10 minutes at room temperature or overnight in the fridge. If leaving overnight in the fridge you may need to add an extra splash of milk in the morning. The texture should resemble a loose porridge.

Nutrition per serving:

Calories 533 | Total carbohydrate 90 g | Sugars 27 g
Fat 12 g | Protein 18 g | Sodium 12 mg

Beetroot and blueberry bircher

A really vibrant breakfast – and recent studies suggest beetroot can help lower blood pressure and boost exercise performance

Now let's be honest here, beetroot juice is an acquired taste at best, but there is lots of good research to suggest it has excellent benefits for us cyclists. The balance of the earthy taste of the beetroot works really well with the sweetness of the blueberries and blueberry yoghurt. Finish off with a teaspoon of honey and a tablespoon of pumpkin seeds.

Serves 1

50 g (2 oz) gluten-free oats

1 tablespoon chia seeds

75 ml (4 ½ tablespoons) milk (can be substituted with a non-dairy milk; unsweetened almond milk works particularly well)

50 g (2 oz) blueberry yoghurt

1 teaspoon concentrated beetroot juice

50 ml (3 tablespoons) beetroot and apple juice (50:50 mix)

60 g (2 ½ oz) frozen blueberries

1 teaspoon honey

1 tablespoon pumpkin seeds

1. Weigh out your dry ingredients (oats and chia seeds) into your breakfast bowl.

2. Add the milk, yoghurt, concentrated beetroot juice and the beetroot and apple juice mix.

3. Stir the frozen blueberries through the mixture.

4. Leave to sit for 10 minutes at room temperature or overnight in the fridge. If leaving overnight in the fridge you may need to add an extra splash of milk in the morning. The texture should resemble a loose porridge.

5. Just before serving, drizzle over the teaspoon of honey and sprinkle on the pumpkin seeds.

Nutrition per serving:
Calories 471 | Total carbohydrate 64 g | Sugars 27 g
Fat 15 g | Protein 18 g | Sodium 9 mg

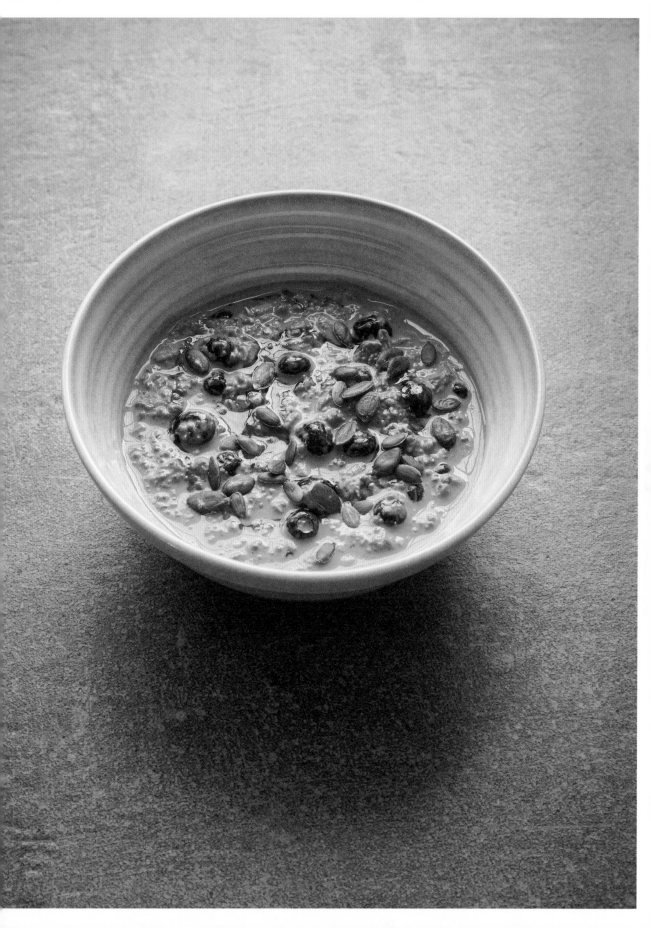

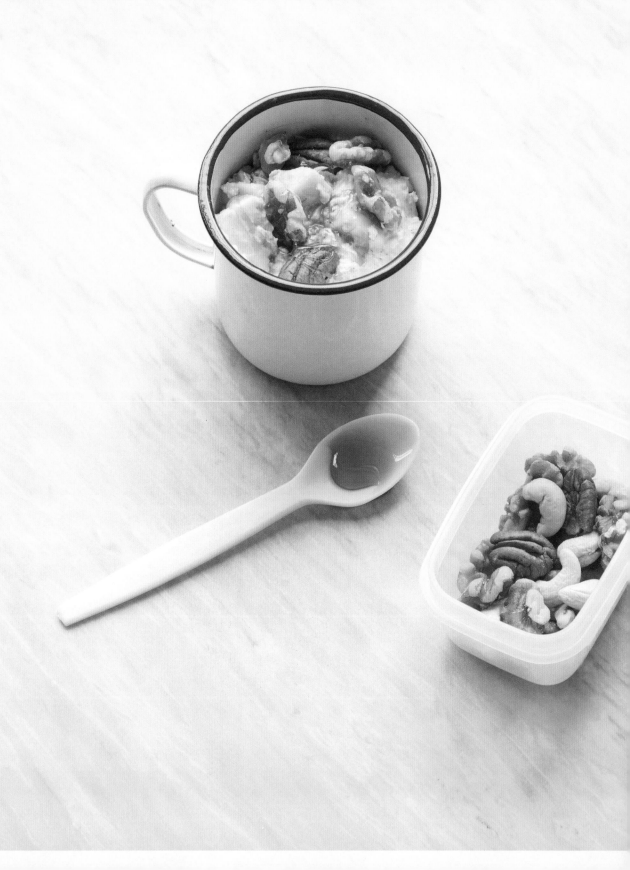

Car boot bircher (peanut butter, soya milk, honey and oats)

This is an on-the-hoof breakfast that is incredibly easy to make when you're travelling

All the ingredients in this recipe are portable and can be kept at room temperature, hence the name. They can be thrown together literally in the back of a car, which is perfect for when you have an early start from a hotel and no access to any cooking facilities.

Serves 1

60 g (2 ½ oz) gluten-free oats (or 1 mug of oats if you don't have any scales with you)

1 tablespoon crunchy nut butter (peanut or almond butter works well)

100 ml (½ cup) soya or rice milk

1 banana, peeled and chopped

1 tablespoon honey

a good handful of mixed nuts such as almonds, cashews or walnuts

1. Dead easy! You can pre-weigh your oats into a lidded plastic container at home or use a mug to estimate while on the road.

2. Add the nut butter, soya milk and chopped banana.

3. Leave to sit for 10 minutes.

4. Top with nuts and honey, and enjoy!

Nutrition per serving:

Calories 646 | Total carbohydrate 82 g | Sugars 31 g
Fat 25 g | Protein 22 g | Sodium 60 mg

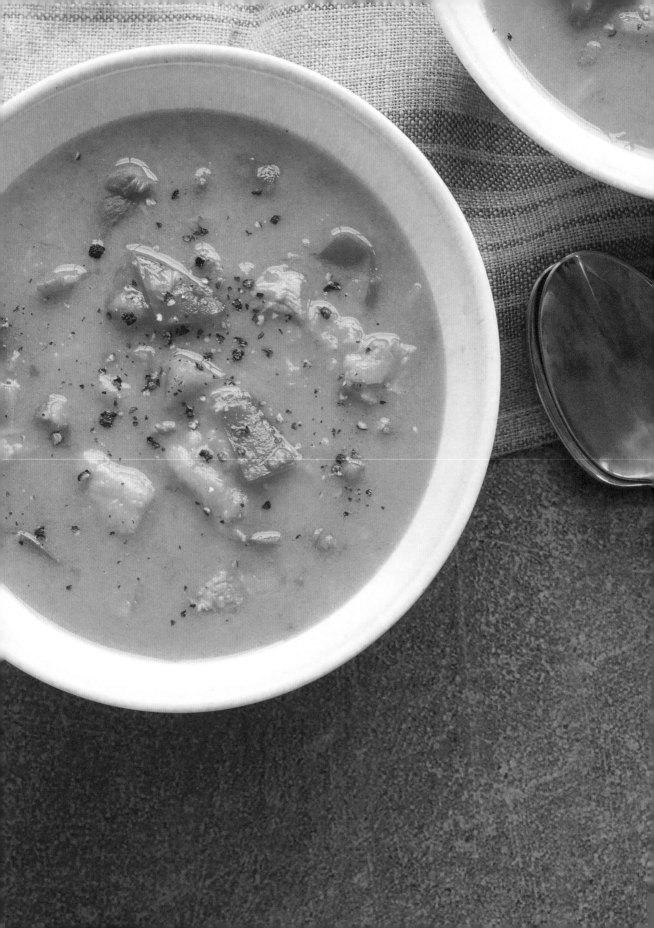

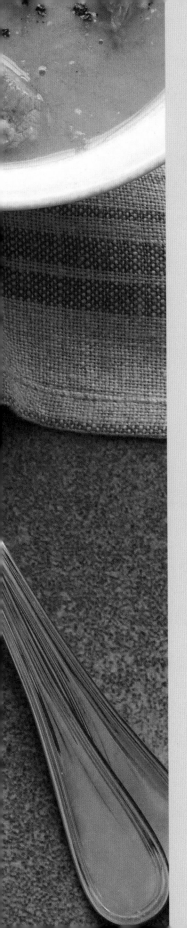

Broths and Soups

A great winter warmer, but easy to prepare and digest any time of year, a soup is ideal cyclist fare. Get your soup technique sorted and you'll open the door to countless brilliantly nutritious and flavoursome meals.

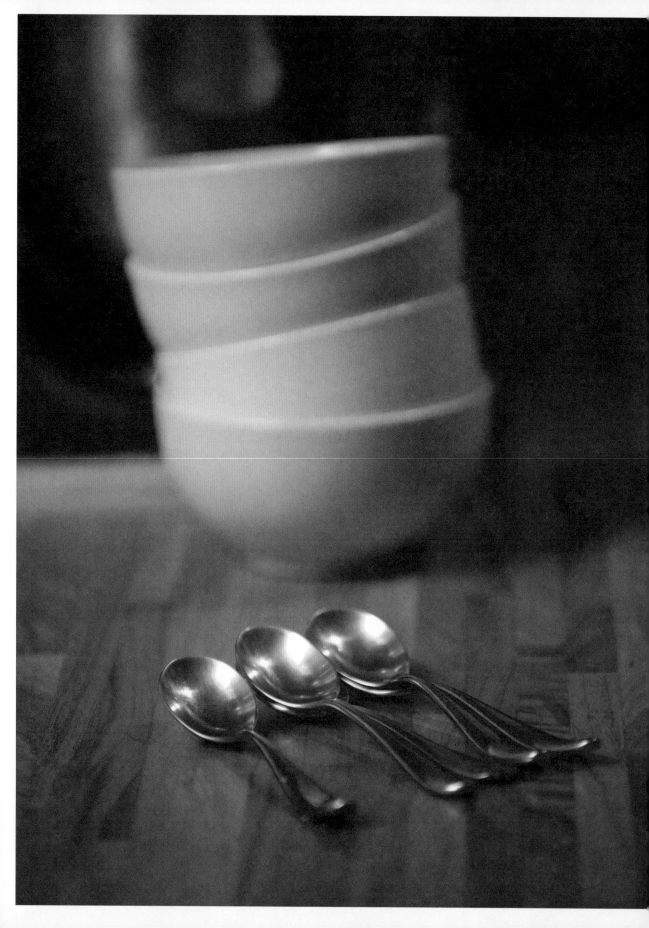

After a chilly winter ride there's little better to come home to than soup. Quickly heated and easily eaten, it can be a fabulous protein-filled recovery meal. But a magic broth can also be valuable as a lunch or evening meal, and a great way of getting extra greens and replenishing carbs, protein and essential minerals – especially when accompanied by a slice of wholemeal bread. Add the fact that it's ideal for pre-cooking and freezing and you've got a meal that could have been designed for cyclists.

The mastery of good soup is a great skill to have. Making good soup is easy, but making great soup isn't that much harder. The key element is the 'caramelisation' or 'sautéing' of the veg, which is critical to getting lots of flavour. Why is this? OK, let's get down to basics. What tastes better, a roast potato or a boiled one? Let's apply the same logic to veg: what's going to taste better, roasted or boiled veg?

Spend a little time getting some colour on your veg and your soup will taste so much better for it. Once you understand the basic principle of getting flavour into veg, then adding a suitable grain or pulse and then a good stock, you will quickly become a soup Jedi!

Buy a decent soup pan, too: it will serve you well. A 25 cm x 12 cm (10 inch x 5 inch) pan is a suitable and versatile size, ideally non-stick. Don't use metal utensils in the bottom of a non-stick pan. Alternatively, opt for a proper cast-iron pan, which should last a lifetime.

Life is too short to make your own stock – you should be out riding your bike or shaving your legs instead! So, use good-quality stock cubes or shop-bought stock. Pretty much any pulse can be added to soups, just amend the cooking time accordingly. When using rice, I prefer brown rice as the texture works really well in soup and reheats perfectly.

Making good soup is easy, but making great soup isn't that much harder. The key element is the 'caramelisation' or 'sautéing' of the veg, which is critical to getting lots of flavour.

Grandmother's chicken soup

Great for lighter training days or as a quick and easy lunch, this soup can easily be made more 'carby' by serving with good-quality bread

This basic soup was a household staple when I was growing up. Easy to prepare using humble ingredients, it can be cooked in one pot in under 30 minutes. It also reheats and freezes really well. Needless to say, my grandmother was not in the habit of using 'fancy' ingredients like pesto! Extra fresh herbs can also be used in place of the pesto.

Makes 6–8 portions

2 tablespoons olive oil

1 white onion, peeled and diced

2 large carrots, trimmed and diced

1 parsnip, trimmed and diced

1 medium swede, trimmed, peeled and diced

1 leek, trimmed and diced

500 g (1 lb 2 oz) skinless chicken breast, diced

100 g (3 ½ oz) brown rice

2000 ml (4 pints) chicken stock (good-quality stock cubes or shop-bought stock)

sea salt and freshly ground black pepper

80 g (3 oz) frozen peas, defrosted

2 tablespoons fresh pesto or a handful of fresh chopped parsley

Nutrition per serving:

Calories 196 | Total carbohydrate 16 g | Sugars 3 g
Fat 7 g | Protein 16 g | Sodium 135 mg

1. Preheat a large saucepan and warm the olive oil. Add the diced vegetables and cook over a medium heat for 4–5 minutes. You are looking to lightly brown the veg (remember, this is key to getting a great flavour).

2. Next, add the diced chicken and cook for a further 4 minutes, stirring every so often.

3. Stir in the brown rice and chicken stock. Bring to the boil and simmer over a low heat for 30–40 minutes until the rice is tender.

4. Adjust the seasoning and add the peas, fresh pesto or chopped parsley at the end to retain freshness. Divide the soup between bowls and serve at once.

5. If freezing, omit the pesto and fresh herbs. Allow the soup to cool fully and freeze in separate 500 g (1 lb 2 oz) portions for convenience. Best kept in the freezer for up to 14 days. Defrost in the fridge for 24 hours, then reheat thoroughly and top with fresh pesto and herbs on serving to retain freshness.

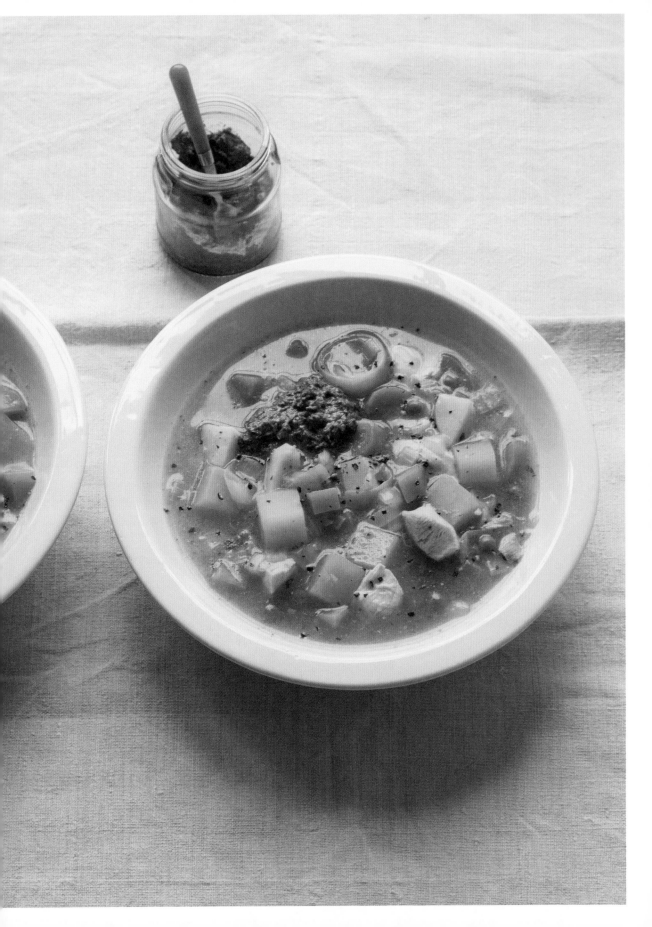

Smoky roast red pepper, chorizo and quinoa soup

Perfect for post-ride refuelling!

Hearty strong flavours and interesting textures make this a post-ride winner. It tastes even better if you make it a day in advance.

Makes 6–8 portions

150 g (5 oz) chorizo, diced (spicy or smoked)

1 onion, peeled and diced

2 red peppers, deseeded and diced

2 medium carrots, trimmed and diced

1 green pepper, deseeded and diced

1 tablespoon chopped garlic

1 tablespoon smoked paprika

1 teaspoon red chilli, deseeded and diced

150 g (5 oz) skinless chicken breast, diced

100 g (3 ½ oz) quinoa

2000 ml (4 pints) chicken stock (good-quality stock cubes or shop-bought stock)

sea salt and freshly ground black pepper

1 small bunch of chopped fresh basil

1. Preheat a large saucepan over a medium heat. Add the chorizo, diced veg and garlic to the pan and stir-fry for 4–5 minutes. The fat from the chorizo will render down, meaning you don't need to add olive oil to cook off the vegetables.

2. Next, add the smoked paprika, chilli and diced chicken. Cook for a further 3 minutes before adding the quinoa and chicken stock. Simmer over a low to medium heat for 20–30 minutes, stirring occasionally to ensure the quinoa does not stick to the bottom of the pan.

3. Adjust the seasoning and then at the last minute stir in the basil. Divide the soup between bowls and serve at once.

Nutrition per serving:

Calories 185 | Total carbohydrate 14 g | Sugars 3 g
Fat 9 g | Protein 11 g | Sodium 750 mg

Vietnamese-style chicken, ginger and coriander broth

This soup is packed with flavour, with a serious ginger kick

This aromatic and flavoursome broth is based around the classic Vietnamese pho. A few years ago I travelled around Vietnam and this was pretty much a staple everywhere I went. It's a healthy and light broth that you can make in advance and works really well on rest days or days when you are looking to have a calorie deficit.

Serves 4

1500 ml (3 pints) chicken stock (good-quality stock cubes or shop-bought stock)

100 g (3 ½ oz) fresh ginger, peeled and roughly chopped

1 small red chilli, deseeded

3 stalks of fresh lemongrass, roughly chopped

500 g (1 lb 2 oz) skinless chicken thighs, diced

1 red pepper, deseeded and sliced

1 yellow pepper, deseeded and sliced

1 green pepper, deseeded and sliced

2 red onions, peeled and sliced

2 heads of pak choi, trimmed and roughly chopped

75 g (3 oz) fresh beansprouts

50 g (2 oz) spring onions, trimmed and finely chopped

1 bunch of fresh coriander, chopped

1 tablespoon fresh grated raw ginger

2 tablespoons Thai fish sauce

1 tablespoon light soy sauce

juice and zest of one lime

Nutrition per serving:

Calories 307 | Total carbohydrate 19 g | Sugars 7 g
Fat 13 g | Protein 27 g | Sodium 501 mg

1. OK, a slightly different method here… Bring the chicken stock to the boil in a large saucepan, then infuse with the chopped ginger, red chilli and lemongrass. Leave to simmer for 15 minutes, then set aside for an hour to cool down.

2. Pass the infused chicken stock through a sieve and return to the pan. Add the diced chicken and simmer over a low heat for 15 minutes. Stir in the sliced peppers and red onions and simmer for a further 5 minutes.

3. Remove from the heat and add the more delicate vegetables, the pak choi and the beansprouts. Stir into the broth and leave for 3–4 minutes.

4. Finally, stir in the spring onions, coriander and ginger, then season with fish sauce, soy sauce and lime juice. The soup should not require any additional seasoning but check it just in case. If you feel it does, add a touch of salt and pepper. Divide between bowls and serve at once.

Variation

For a slightly more filling broth, add some cooked rice noodles at the same time as you add the peppers. You can easily replace the chicken with fish or shellfish, just adjust the cooking times accordingly. Add the fish or shellfish when you add the peppers and onions.

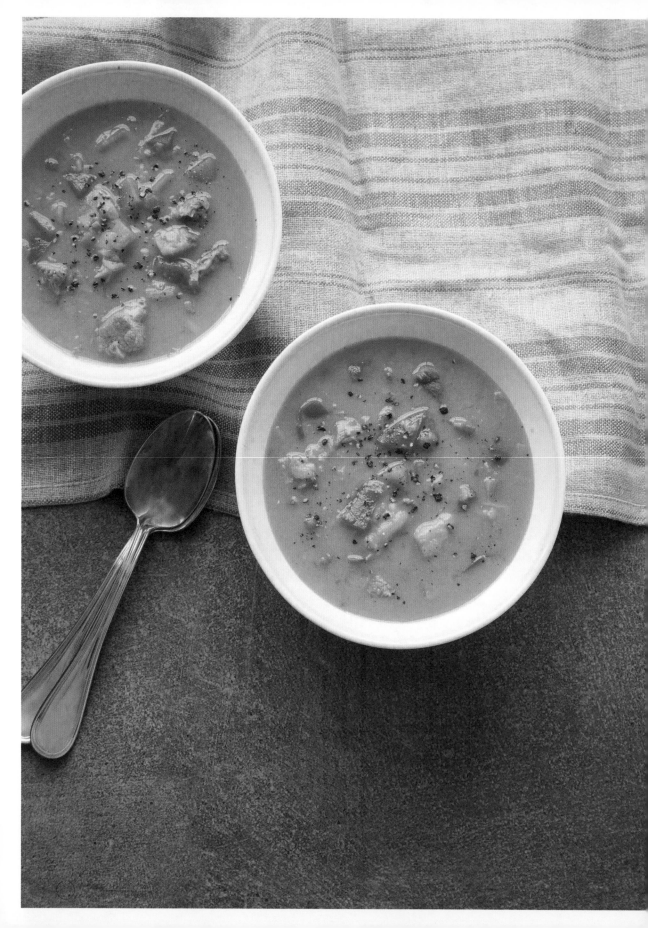

Roast lamb, harissa and red lentil soup

A pretty full-on soup, this one – good for a post-long ride lunch. Just stick it all in the slow cooker and ride your bike for three hours. Simple!

A proper meal in a bowl, this soup has been created for the slow cooker, but the more time you take to cook it, the better. If you don't own a slow cooker, it can easily be cooked in a large saucepan – just make sure you stir it regularly or the lentils will catch on the base of the pan. When cooking in a pan, add 500 ml (2 cups) of water as the liquid will reduce. For a vegan soup, simply replace the lamb with 500 g (1 lb 2 oz) diced butternut squash and use vegetable stock.

Serves 6

2 tablespoons olive oil

500 g (1 lb 2 oz) diced lamb shoulder

2 teaspoons Harissa paste

1 teaspoon crushed coriander seeds

1 teaspoon paprika

1 teaspoon dried turmeric

1 large onion, peeled and diced

2 carrots, trimmed and diced

2 red peppers, deseeded and diced

1 large sweet potato, peeled and diced

100 g (3 ½ oz) red lentils

1500 ml (3 pints) chicken or vegetable stock (good-quality stock cubes or shop-bought stock)

400 ml (2 cups) coconut milk

sea salt and freshly ground black pepper

Nutrition per serving:
Calories 322 | Total carbohydrate 17 g | Sugars 5 g | Fat 20 g
Protein 18 g | Sodium 215 mg

1. It's best to sear the lamb and all the vegetables first before transferring to the slow cooker – you will get more flavour this way. Preheat a large saucepan, add the olive oil and sear the lamb over high heat for 5–7 minutes. Stir in the Harissa paste, coriander seeds, paprika and turmeric. Cook for a further 2 minutes, then transfer to the slow cooker. At this point, turn on the slow cooker to heat up – it will take a few minutes.

2. Use the same pan to colour off the veg: add the onion, carrots, peppers and sweet potato to the same saucepan and cook over a medium heat for 4–5 minutes. Stir in the red lentils and add everything to the lamb mix in the slow cooker.

3. In the same pan again, heat the stock and add the coconut milk, stirring. Transfer to the pre-heated slow cooker and place on a low heat with the lid on for 3 hours or medium heat for 1 hour 30 minutes. Once the lentils are soft and the lamb is tender, adjust the seasoning and serve at once in bowls.

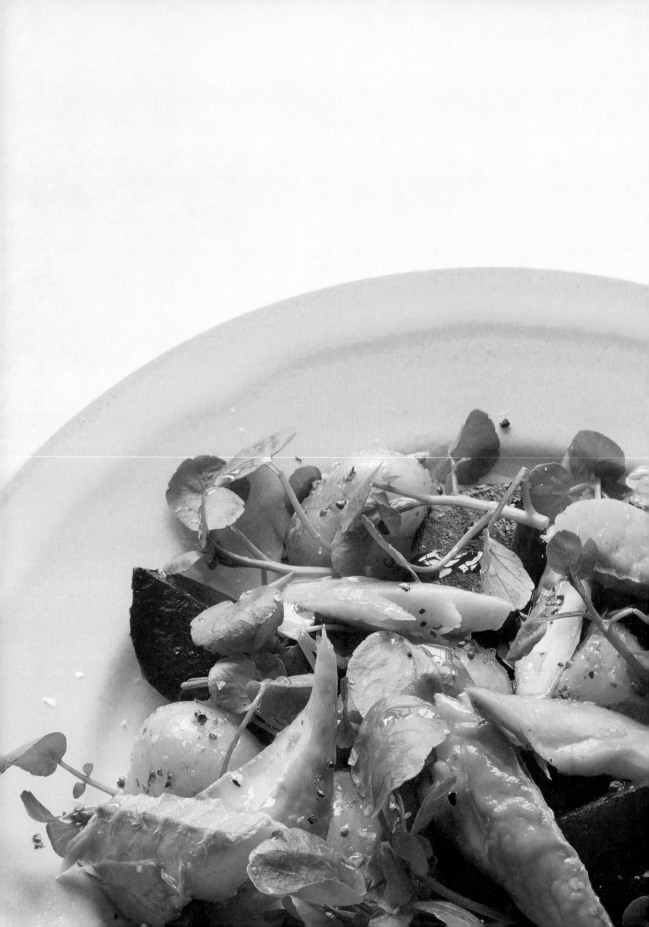

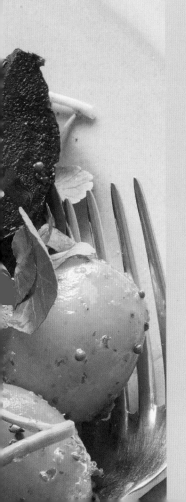

Main Meals

When we sit down to eat, what are cyclists looking for in a meal? Carbs, protein, vitamins? Sure, all that, but like everyone else we want it to look good and taste great. These main meal ideas provide all the nutrition you need along with a ton of flavour.

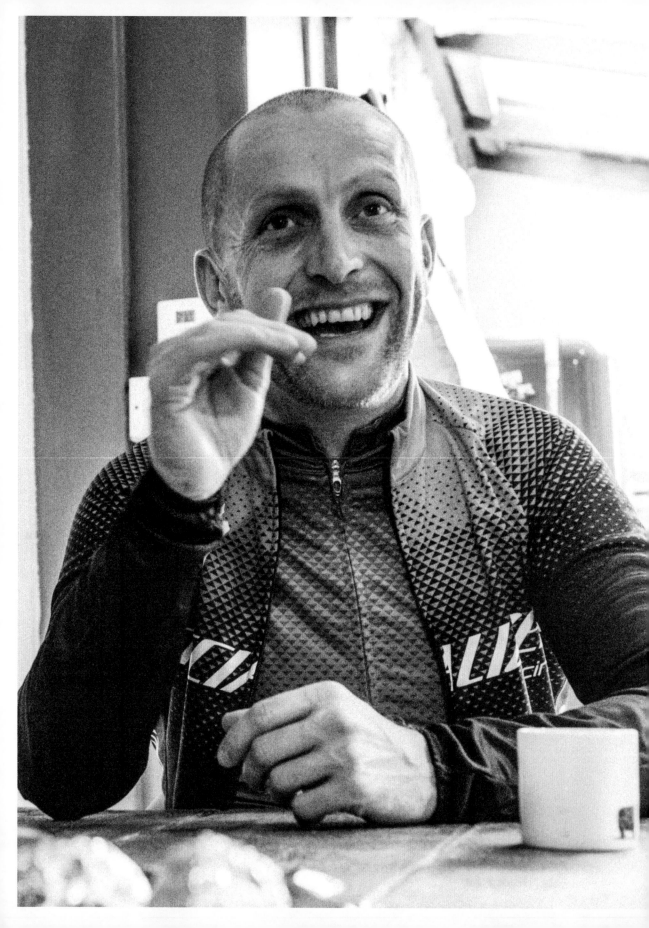

Eating for optimum performance doesn't mean eating boring or bland food; it means exactly the opposite. Eating the same meal again and again won't provide a balance of nutrients. On the other hand, a little consideration of what your body needs will lead to you consuming a range of texture and flavours, improving your cooking skills and discovering new ingredients and recipes.

While you are looking to achieve a nutritional balance in your diet, not every meal needs to be a finely honed mix of carbs, protein and fats. It is fine to balance nutrients out over the week. Also consider what your body requires: a carbohydrate-heavy meal is not necessary if you are not training hard or racing.

My experience of high-performance athletes – even those who really like their food – is that they have neither the energy nor inclination to spend hours in the kitchen. The recipes included here all involve minimal preparation, a maximum cooking time of 30 minutes and use one or two pans.

What I would advise is to be adventurous. Ingredients are interchangeable. You can use pretty much any form of protein you choose; it does not matter much if you substitute chicken for turkey or vice versa. Red meat might come down to what you can get and what your budget allows. And remember, pulses are a great source of protein too – you don't need meat with every meal.

Finally, beware fads. Maybe there is a magic diet somewhere out there that will solve all our problems, but a balanced diet is the only one that's stood the test of time. Similarly, superfood ingredients won't save the universe: they might be packed full of goodness, but so are chickpeas, eggs and oats.

My experience of high-performance athletes – even those who really like their food – is that they have neither the energy nor inclination to spend hours in the kitchen.

Turkey mince chilli with coriander and lime guacamole

Turkey is an excellent lean protein source and is a great alternative to minced beef when you want to keep the fat and calorie content down.

This meal can be thrown together in no time and also freezes really well, so it's the perfect back-up when you're time poor. It's OK to use 'lazy' chilli and garlic – a pre-prepared product like this saves a lot of faffing around. All the major supermarkets sell kidney beans and mixed beans in a mildly spicy tomato-based sauce, so feel free to use these. Low in fat, high in protein and fibre, this works really well when served with baked sweet potatoes.

Serves 4–6

1 tablespoon olive oil

500 g (1 lb 2 oz) turkey mince

1 teaspoon each deseeded chopped red and green chillies

1 teaspoon 'lazy' chopped garlic

1 large red onion, peeled and diced

3 peppers, deseeded and diced

1 x tin taco bean mix (395 g / 14 oz)

1 x tin kidney beans (395 g / 14 oz)

1 x tin sweetcorn (198 g / 7 oz)

500 g (1 lb 2 oz) chopped plum tomatoes

3 chopped fresh tomatoes

Guacamole

2 large ripe avocado, peeled and pitted

1 tablespoon extra virgin olive oil

1 teaspoon deseeded chopped green chilli

1 teaspoon lime juice

1 tablespoon chopped fresh coriander

10 crushed coriander seeds

sea salt and freshly ground black pepper

1. Make the guacamole in advance. Place all the ingredients in a food processor and blend until smooth. Transfer to a bowl, cover and refrigerate. Keeps well for up to 2–3 hours; any longer and you are at risk of it going brown.

2. Preheat a large saucepan, add the olive oil and fry the turkey mince for 4–5 minutes over a medium heat until lightly browned. Break down any chunks of mince with a wooden spoon as it cooks. Add the chillies, garlic, onion and peppers. Fry for a further 3–4 minutes, stirring occasionally.

3. The next stage is to add the taco bean mix, kidney beans, sweetcorn and chopped plum tomatoes. Simmer gently for about 20 minutes.

4. Season well and sprinkle with chopped fresh tomato. Serve with the guacamole.

Nutrition per serving:
Calories 341 | Total carbohydrate 23 g | Sugars 12 g | Fat 15 g
Protein 29 g | Sodium 268 g

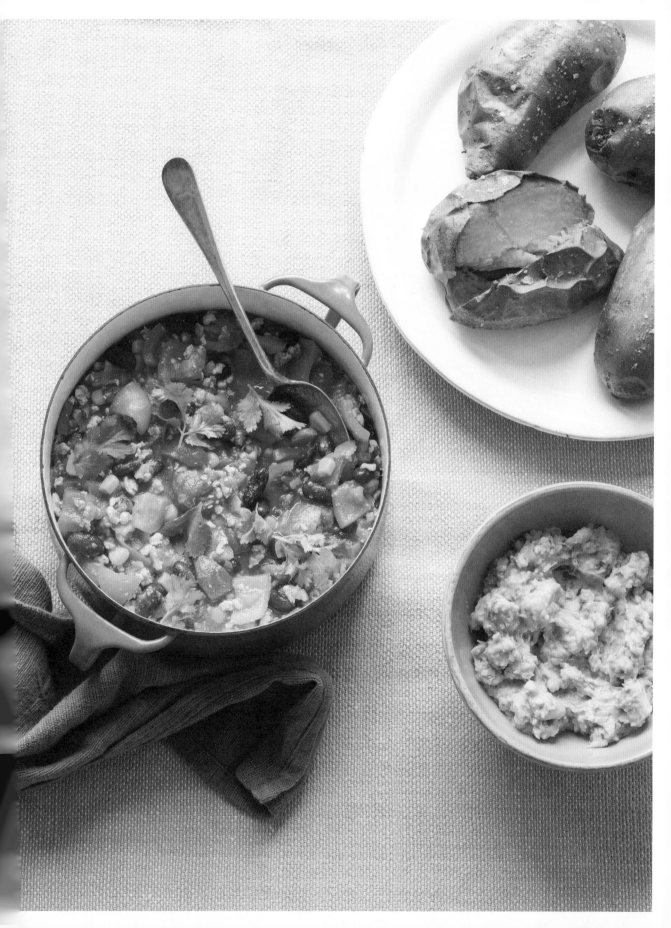

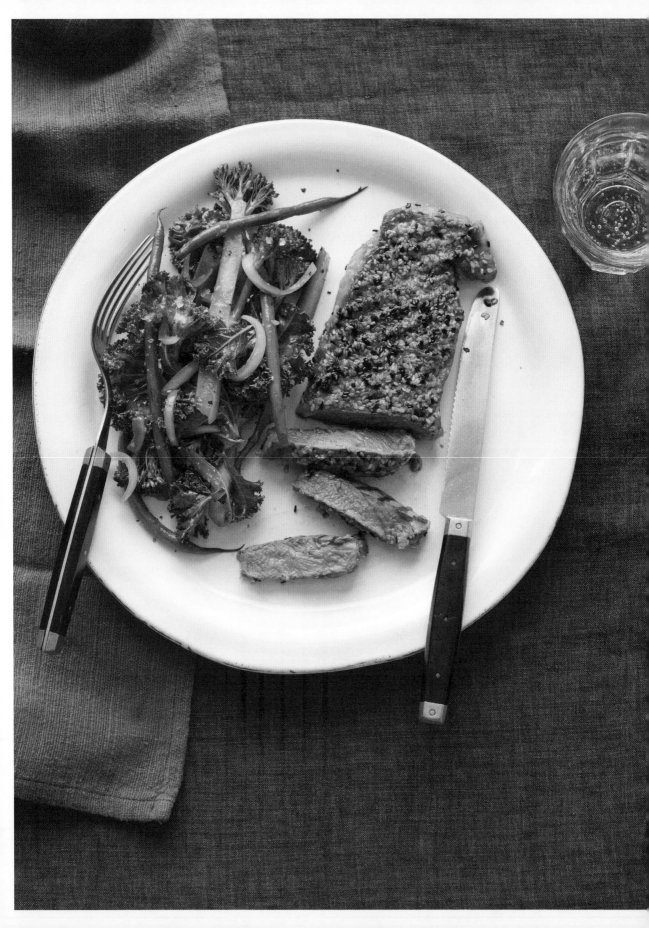

Grilled sesame seed steak with greens and soy sauce

Steak has an important place on the cyclist's menu. If you fancy some carbs, this works really well with rice or rice noodles

Red meat contains haem iron, which is more easily absorbed than the non-haem iron found in plant sources. Good iron levels are essential as iron deficiency leads to fatigue and an impairment of your cycling performance. The cut of steak is a very personal choice. Fillet is extremely tender but expensive. Rump steak has a much firmer texture and great flavour, but can be tricky to cook. Rib-eye is probably the 'chef's choice', being a tender piece of meat and full of flavour, but it usually contains more fat. The safest bet is sirloin – firm, flavoursome and easy to cook.

Serves 2

1 teaspoon black sesame seeds

1 tablespoon white sesame seeds

sea salt and freshly ground black pepper

2 steaks (allow 190–200 g / 6 ½–7 oz per person)

1 teaspoon olive oil

1 tablespoon soy sauce

1 tablespoon coconut oil

1 white onion, peeled and sliced

1 tablespoon fresh grated ginger

1 tablespoon chopped garlic

good selection of chopped greens: pak choi, mangetouts, spinach, kale, green beans, broccoli

1 teaspoon Thai fish sauce

1 tablespoon Teriyaki sauce

1 teaspoon sesame oil

Nutrition per serving:

Calories 552 | Total carbohydrate 25 g | Sugars 10 g
Fat 22 g | Protein 75 g | Sodium 834 mg

1. Preheat a grill pan and a large sauté pan – we are going to cook two things at once!

2. In a bowl, mix together the black and white sesame seeds. Add a good pinch of sea salt and some freshly ground black pepper. Place the steaks on a plate and sprinkle the seed mixture over the top.

3. Heat the olive oil in the grill pan and sear the steak over a high heat for 2 minutes each side. At the last minute add the soy sauce to the pan to glaze the steaks. Remove the steaks from the pan, transfer to a warmed plate and allow to rest for 3–4 minutes.

4. Heat the coconut oil in the sauté pan and stir-fry the onion over a high heat for 1 minute. Add the fresh ginger and garlic and cook for a further 2 minutes.

5. Next, add the mixed greens. Continue cooking over a high heat for a further 2 minutes (you want the veg to be crunchy and have some bite to it). Finish off by adding the fish and Teriyaki sauces and sesame oil. Slice the steak and serve with the greens.

Chicken sausages with spicy bean cassoulet and crispy polenta

This bean cassoulet dish is high in protein and fibre – a nod to my classical training in French cuisine reinvented for cyclists. Classic flavours never go out of fashion!

Chicken sausages are a bit of a revelation for me. We tend to associate sausages with cooked breakfasts and not as part of a healthy main meal. Most supermarkets sell chicken sausages, but if you have a good local butcher go there. Pre-cooked polenta is available in most supermarkets.

Serves 2

100 g (3 ½ oz) spicy chorizo, diced

100 g (3 ½ oz) lean smoked bacon, chopped

1 red pepper, deseeded and diced

1 yellow pepper, deseeded and diced

1 white onion, peeled and diced

1 teaspoon 'lazy' chopped garlic

1 teaspoon deseeded and diced red chilli

1 tin butter beans (240 g / 9 oz drained weight)

1 tin baked beans (415 g / 14 oz)

200 ml (¾ cup) chicken stock (good-quality stock cubes or shop-bought stock)

sea salt and freshly ground black pepper

12 large basil leaves, finely sliced

6 chicken sausages (look for good-quality ones from your local butcher or supermarket)

1 teaspoon olive oil

250 g (9 oz) pre-cooked polenta

25 g (1 oz) butter, melted

1. To make the cassoulet mix, place the chorizo and bacon in a large saucepan. Set over a medium heat and fry for 4–5 minutes until the fat has rendered down from the chorizo and the bacon has started to cook. Add the peppers, onion, garlic and chilli; fry for a further 4 minutes.

2. Stir in the butter beans, baked beans and chicken stock. Simmer for 15 minutes over a low heat. Adjust the seasoning and stir in the basil.

3. While the cassoulet is cooking, preheat the grill to medium heat and, using a pastry brush, brush the sausages with the olive oil. Cut the pre-cooked polenta into 2–3 cm slices and brush with melted butter. Grill the sausages and polenta for 8–10 minutes, turning two or three times to ensure they cook evenly.

4. Serve the sausages and polenta with the cassoulet.

Nutrition per serving:

Calories 990 | Total carbohydrate 76 g | Sugars 15 g
Fat 38 g | Protein 75 g | Sodium 4906 mg

Lazy cyclist's salad

This is quite possibly the laziest meal out there, but the balance of ingredients here gives you pretty much everything you need from a nutritional perspective

We all have days when we don't have time to cook, or we don't have anything in the house. All of the ingredients here can be picked up at any mini supermarket and thrown together in less than five minutes as a perfect quick lunch or dinner. This sort of meal has got me out of jail more than once!

Serves 2

250 g (9 oz) pre-cooked quinoa

200 g (7 oz) cucumber, chopped

1 large ripe avocado, peeled, pitted and chopped

100 g (3 ½ oz) chopped spring greens or gem lettuce

3 tablespoons hummus

150 g (5 oz) cold smoked salmon

2 tablespoons pumpkin seeds

1. Simply place the quinoa, chopped cucumber, chunks of avocado and spring greens or lettuce in a large bowl, and stir in the hummus.

2. Serve in salad bowls topped with the smoked salmon and pumpkin seeds. This salad also works really well with grilled chicken or tinned tuna instead of the salmon.

Nutrition per serving:

Calories 626 | Total carbohydrate 51 g | Sugars 5 g
Fat 35 g | Protein 31 g | Sodium 105 mg

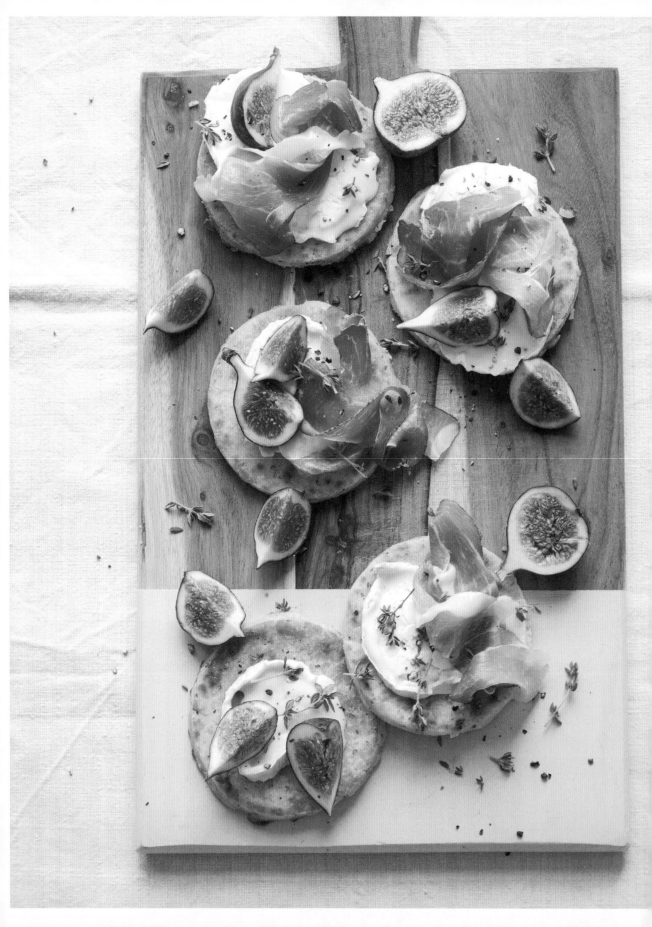

High-protein mini flatbreads

During training, race and rest days, the professionals use protein to promote recovery and optimal body composition

OK, this one is a bit of a faff, but so worth it! Extremely tasty, high in protein and carbohydrate, these flatbreads have a fantastic texture and can be made up in advance and then put through the oven last minute. Of all the dishes I eat on a regular basis this is up there as one of my favourites. Serve with a big green salad and salted tomatoes. With the toppings, you can freestyle it and go with whatever you like.

Makes 9 (enough for 2–3 depending on appetite)

3 tablespoons extra virgin olive oil

185 g (6 ½ oz) full-fat Greek yoghurt

8 sprigs fresh rosemary, finely chopped

a good pinch of sea salt

300 g (11 oz) gluten-free self-raising flour (extra for shaping)

1 tablespoon olive oil for cooking

a big green salad and salted tomatoes (drizzle with olive oil and season), best served at room temperature

Some simple topping suggestions

- Pesto, grilled skinless chicken, rocket, Parmesan shavings and pine nuts

- Parma ham, goat's cheese and caramelised red onions

- Bacon, cheese (mozzarella or a strong cheddar will work well here, depending on personal preference) and sliced tomato

- Sautéed red peppers, chorizo and Manchego

1. Preheat the oven to 190°C/375°F/Gas 5.

2. In a mixing bowl combine the extra virgin olive oil, yoghurt, rosemary and sea salt. Gradually incorporate the flour and knead to a smooth dough.

3. On a floured surface, shape the dough with your hands into a sausage and cut into 9 evenly sized pieces. Press each piece into a disc about 5 mm (¼ inch) thick (freehand or use a pastry cutter to guide you).

4. Heat a little of the olive oil in a griddle or frying pan. Cook each flatbread for 2 minutes on each side until slightly browned (you will be able to do a few at a time). Arrange on a non-stick baking tray and finish off with your choice of topping. Bake for 8–10 minutes and then serve with a green salad and salted tomatoes.

Nutrition per serving:

Calories 603 | Total carbohydrate 83 g | Sugars 1 g | Fat 27 g
Protein 7 g | Sodium 481 mg

Hookers' pasta – or in fancy Italian *'pasta puttanesca'*

When you are looking to refuel at lunchtime, go for carbs and quality protein – this pasta dish is ideal

There's a time and a place for a fix of tasty pasta! All the ingredients used here are essentially store cupboard items. This simple dish can be made in sub-10 minutes, which in my eyes makes it a winner.

Serves 2

200 g (7 oz) spaghetti

2 tablespoons olive oil

3 garlic cloves, peeled and chopped

1 small red chilli, deseeded and finely chopped

75 g (3 oz) salted anchovies, chopped

500 g (1 lb 2 oz) passata

200 g (7 oz) good-quality pitted black olives or green anchovy stuffed olives

3 tablespoons chopped capers

small bunch of fresh basil

50 g (2 oz) Parmesan, grated

1. Put a large saucepan of salted water on to boil. Once boiling, get your spaghetti on! Reduce to a simmer and cook according to the instructions on the packet. Remember, dried pasta takes longer than fresh, so work out timings for the pasta and sauce first.

2. Heat the olive oil in a sauté pan and fry the garlic, chilli and anchovies in the oil over a low heat for 2–3 minutes. Stir in the passata, olives and capers; simmer gently until the pasta is cooked.

3. Strain the spaghetti and stir into the sauce. Transfer to plates or bowls and finish off with a scattering of torn fresh basil and grated Parmesan.

Nutrition per serving:

Calories 879 | Total carbohydrate 93 g | Sugars 8 g | Fat 41 g
Protein 35 g | Sodium 3173 mg

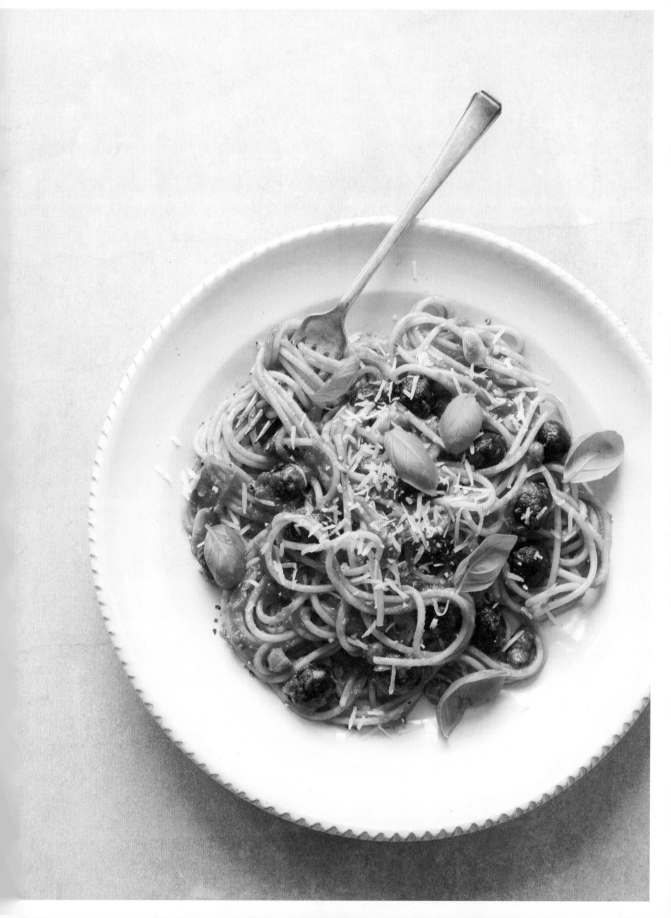

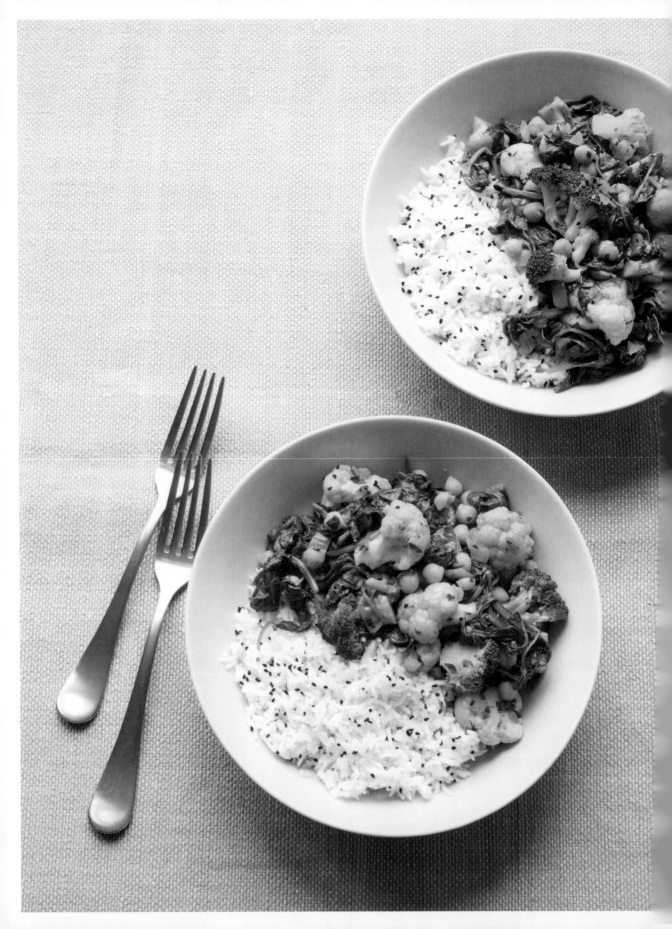

Tikka-spiced cauliflower, broccoli and chickpea curry

A low-fat, high flavour, inexpensive vegan curry… well I never!

The quality of the curry powder goes a long way to determining how well this dish turns out, so choose a good one. Also, quick cooking for this dish, please – if you cook it slow and long, all the veg becomes stewed and breaks down into mush, which is simply not cool! For all you carnivores out there, you can easily add diced chicken breast with the onions.

Serves 2–3

1 teaspooon coconut oil

1 onion, peeled and chopped

2 tablespoons tikka curry powder

1 teaspoon fresh grated turmeric (fresh is best, but dried can be substituted)

300 g (11 oz) cauliflower, finely chopped

200 g (7 oz) broccoli, finely chopped

1 tin (215 g / 7 ½ oz drained weight) cooked chickpeas or butter beans

300 ml (1 ¼ cups) vegetable stock (good-quality stock cubes or shop-bought stock)

1 large bag (500 g / 1 lb 2 oz) baby spinach leaves

1 bunch of fresh coriander

1 tablespoon black onion seeds

sea salt and freshly ground black pepper

1. In a large high-sided sauté pan, heat the coconut oil. Fry the chopped onion in the oil over a medium heat for 2–3 minutes until lightly coloured.

2. Stir in the tikka curry powder and turmeric and cook for a further 2 minutes.

3. Next up is the cauliflower and broccoli: add these to the onion mix and cook over a medium heat for 2–3 minutes.

4. Strain off the chickpeas or butter beans and add to the spiced vegetable mix. Stir in the vegetable stock and cook for 15 minutes over a medium to high heat. Once the liquid is reduced by a third, stir in the baby spinach leaves, fresh coriander and black onion seeds. Correct the seasoning and enjoy!

Nutrition per serving:

Calories 225 | Total carbohydrate 31 g | Sugars 6 g | Fat 5 g
Protein 14 g | Sodium 239 mg

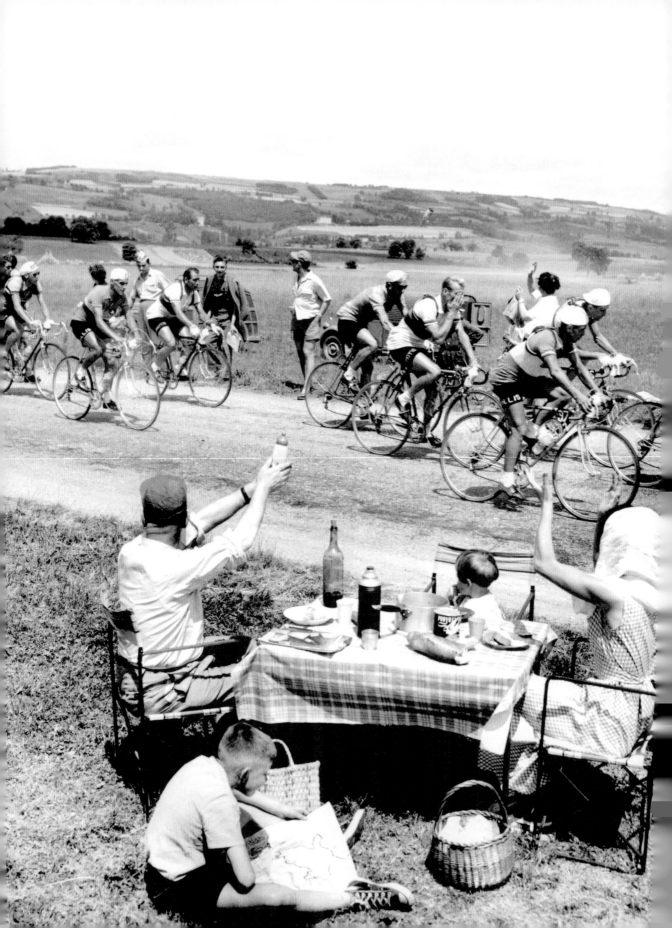

On the Go

You can follow a dietary plan strictly, provide your body with the right nutrients and eat to a schedule, but the rules change again the moment you get on the bike.

Fuelling a tough ride of an hour or more needs preparation and consideration. Here's the conundrum: your body can only store glycogen (the body's source of energy) for a maximum of 90 minutes' riding at high pace. If you carry on after that without taking on more fuel you will lose energy fast or, as cyclists say, 'bonk' or 'hit the wall'. Regular refuelling is therefore necessary, but that can be tricky when you are riding flat out, on high alert for obstacles and escapees, or simply don't feel like eating.

Enjoying a prime view, a French family eat and drink at a table by the roadside during the 1954 Tour de France. Riders don't have this luxury and have to eat smartly on the go.

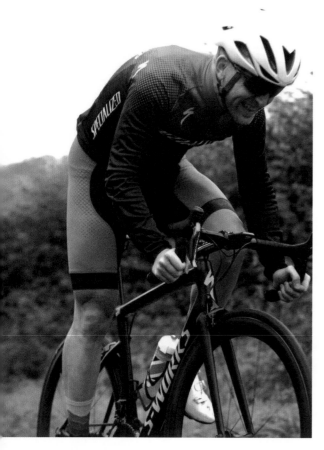

Regular refuelling and rehydration can be tricky when you are riding flat out or simply don't feel like eating.

Just as your training rides are crucial to fitness, they are also key to conditioning the digestive system. Eat properly on your training rides and you can not only assess what you need to consume, but also train your gut to digest on the go and speed up the absorption rate of nutrients into the bloodstream. The bottom line is that as a rule of thumb you will need to take on board around 1 g of carbohydrates per kilo of body weight each hour, but on top of that you need to consider the weight and effect of the food you are carrying, whether it is portable or will disintegrate in your pocket, and, just as importantly, whether you can face eating it when the time comes.

On a long ride you – and your digestive system – are going to get pretty sick of bars and gels. Riders call it 'flavour fatigue' when they reach the limit of the amount of sweet foods and sickly gels they can stomach. The ideal musette (or back-pocket food stash) will contain a variety of sweet and savoury items and a mix of fast and slow energy-releasing carbs, ranging from sliced-up fruit, flapjacks and gels to beef biltong, boiled potatoes and rice cakes, as well as light snacks, such as courgette muffins and small sandwiches made from wholewheat bread. Some also claim that a mix of glucose (from carbohydrates) and fructose (from fruit and veg) can increase oxidation by as much as 50 per cent, another reason to vary the sort of snacks you're taking with you on a ride.

Hydration is vital to the digestion of nutrients. How much fluid to consume depends on the individual and the weather conditions. A long ride should result in no more than around two per cent loss in body weight, so weigh yourself before and after training rides. If you lose more than two pounds through sweat, consider increasing your fluid intake. Drink little and often, switching between water and electrolytes – depending on the weather conditions, you should be getting through one 750-ml bidon (water bottle) every hour.

Planning plays a role too. Consider your post-race recovery food. Make sure a smoothie or any other snacks will be ready to hand when you finish riding and prepare any meal as much as possible. You will be grateful not to have to do it when you are exhausted from a ride. Three to four hours before you ride have a substantial breakfast (*see also* p. 40) and make sure you are fully hydrated, then start out as you mean to continue: after 20 minutes begin drinking and eating small amounts at regular intervals. Some riders even set a reminder alarm to sound every 20 minutes.

The nature of the ride will also dictate what and when you consume. Eat any slow-release items – sandwiches or bananas – early on. Then remain aware of what effort you are putting in and fuel appropriately. Is the peloton setting a high pace? Is it a particularly gruelling climb or are you about to embark on an escape? Fuel up for any extra demands on the body or periods when you know you will be unable to eat or drink. As you enter the last hour of the ride, switch to gels, caffeine or sugary drinks – these will give you a quick energy boost when your body is tired and under stress.

Preparation Rules

- Use training sessions to help decide what you need and like to eat on a ride.
- Ensure you have eaten well and hydrated properly in the hours before a long ride.
- Select your musette (back-pocket food stash) from a variety of sweet and savoury foods, gels and drinks.
- Prepare your recovery food before setting off.
- Be clear about what and when you might receive in supplies from support or a feeding station.
- Fuel regularly (even when you don't feel hungry or thirsty) and strategically.
- Re-fuel as soon as possible after you complete the ride.

Suggested On-the-go Foods

- Bananas
- Rice cakes
- Homemade energy bars (*see* p. 154)
- Small peanut butter or jam sandwiches
- Muffins or banana bread (*see* pp. 177–178)
- Brownies or flapjacks (*see* pp. 155, 175).

'Scottish' paella

An easy-to-cook, one-pan dinner that's ideal for a post-ride recovery and just as good the next day for lunch

OK, so why Scottish? Isn't paella traditionally a Spanish dish? Well, we all know Scottish people like me are allegedly 'careful' with money, so here we are using turmeric as opposed to expensive saffron to flavour the rice. Turmeric has performance benefits for cyclists as it is a natural anti-inflammatory. With starchy carbs and high protein levels, this recipe is good for a pre-race meal or the night before a hard session or a long day in the saddle. It also reheats really well, meaning any leftovers can be used for a quick and easy post-ride refuel.

Serves 2–3

100 g (3 ½ oz) smoked chorizo, diced

1 red pepper, deseeded and diced

1 yellow pepper, deseeded and diced

1 onion, peeled and diced

200 g (7 oz) skinless chicken breast, diced

2 teaspoons dried turmeric

200 g (7 oz) Arborio (risotto) rice

650 ml (2 ½ cups) chicken or vegetable stock (good-quality stock cubes or shop-bought stock)

200 g (7 oz) diced firm fish (such as salmon, haddock or halibut, or shelled raw prawns)

100 g (3 ½ oz) frozen peas, defrosted

sea salt and freshly ground black pepper

a pinch of smoked paprika

Nutrition per serving:
Calories 616 | Total carbohydrate 70 g | Sugars 6 g | Fat 17 g
Protein 46 g | Sodium 397 mg

1. Start by preheating a large sauté pan. Add the chorizo to the dry pan and cook over a medium heat for 2–3 minutes until some of the fat has rendered down.

2. Add the peppers and onion to the pan and continue cooking for 3–4 minutes over a medium heat. There should be enough oil from the chorizo, meaning you don't need to add any extra oil to the pan.

3. Now, stir in the chicken and turmeric. Cook for a further 3 minutes before adding the risotto rice and stock. Simmer gently for about 18 minutes until the liquid has been absorbed and rice is tender; depending on the rice and how hard you cook the risotto, you might need to add a touch more liquid, so keep an eye on it.

4. Next, add the diced raw fish or prawns and the peas. Cook gently for a further 2–3 minutes, then remove from the heat and allow to sit for a few minutes for the rice to fluff up. Finally, adjust the seasoning with sea salt, freshly ground black pepper and smoked paprika and you are there!

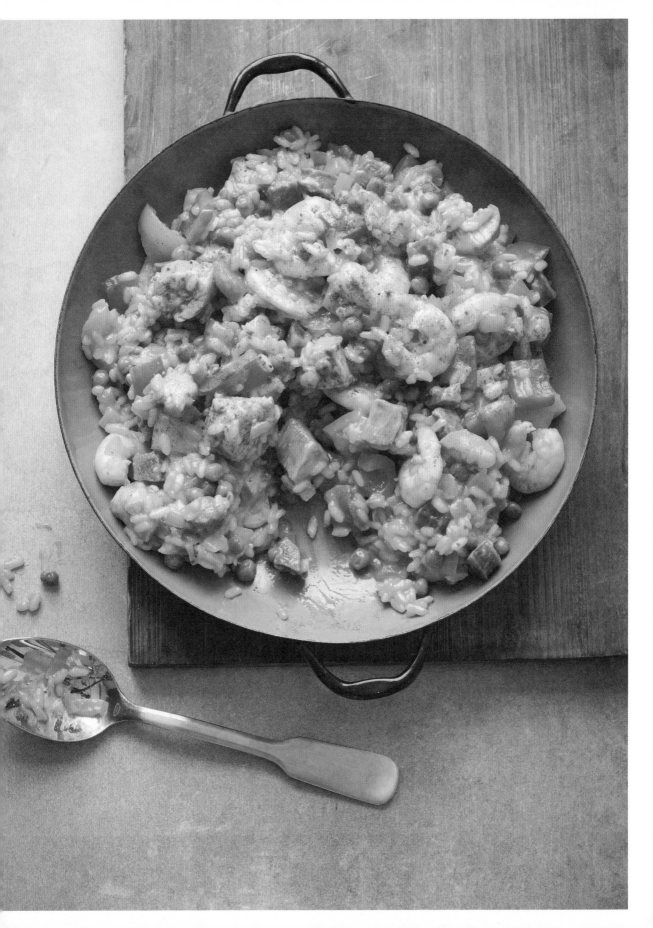

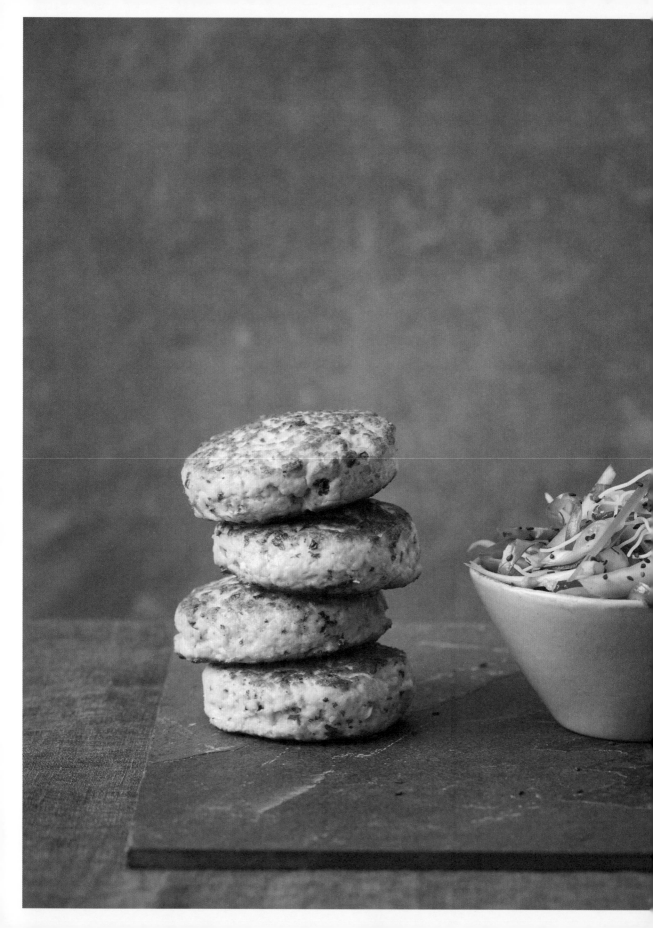

Asian-style turkey burgers

Sweet, spicy and salty... perfect refuelling!

Turkey mince is an excellent low-fat source of protein and amino acids. I try to incorporate it into weekly food plans for all my athletes. The raw veg slaw has a lovely texture – a great contrast to the burgers. 'Lazy' chilli, garlic and ginger comes pre-chopped and is available in jars from most supermarkets.

Serves 2–4 (makes 4 x 125 g / 4 oz burgers)

500 g (1 lb 2 oz) turkey mince (breast meat)

1 tablespoon 'lazy' chilli

1 tablespoon 'lazy' garlic

1 tablespoon 'lazy' ginger

1 tablespoon rice flour or gluten-free flour

1 tablespoon sesame seeds

1 egg

2 tablespoons finely chopped fresh coriander

sea salt and freshly ground black pepper

1 tablespoon olive oil

Asian slaw

100 g (3 ½ oz) pre-cooked fine rice noodles

1 tablespoon sesame oil

2 tablespoons gluten-free soy sauce

2 tablespoons Thai fish sauce

2 tablespoons sweet chilli sauce

1 small red chilli, deseeded and diced

juice of 1 fresh lime

2 carrots, trimmed and grated

1 large courgette, trimmed and grated

1 red onion, peeled and finely sliced

1 red pepper, deseeded and sliced

1 green pepper, deseeded and sliced

1 head of pak choi, sliced

small bunch of spring onions, trimmed and finely chopped

3 tablespoons chopped fresh coriander

sea salt and freshly ground black pepper

1 teaspoon black sesame seeds, to serve

1. Start by making the Asian slaw. Mix together in a bowl all the ingredients apart from the sesame seeds, cover and place in the fridge for 15 minutes. Before serving, check the seasoning and then sprinkle over the black sesame seeds.

2. To make the burgers, combine the turkey mince with all the remaining ingredients apart from the olive oil, ensuring the flour and egg are incorporated well before seasoning. The best way to do this job is to mix everything with your hands – just wash them thoroughly afterwards.

3. To cook the burgers, preheat an oven to 190°C/375°F/Gas 5. Meanwhile, divide the burger mix into four. Preheat a non-stick pan with an ovenproof handle and add the olive oil. Place a 90-mm (3.5 inch) pastry cutter (if you are feeling flash) in the pan. Spoon a quarter of the burger mix into the cutter, press down well and remove the cutter to leave a neat patty. Repeat the shaping process three more times. If you don't have a pastry cutter, don't worry – just shape the mixture into rustic burger patties with your hands.

4. Lightly colour the burgers for 2 minutes on each side, then place the pan in the preheated oven for 10–12 minutes. (If you don't have an ovenproof pan, arrange the burgers on a non-stick baking tray instead).

5. Check the burgers are cooked through (just cut into one with a knife and make sure they are piping hot and there's no raw meat inside), then serve with the Asian slaw.

Nutrition per serving:

Calories 434 | Total carbohydrate 30 g | Sugars 11 g | Fat 13 g
Protein 50 g | Sodium 702 mg

Glazed gnocchi with spinach, broccoli, chicken and tarragon

This gnocchi bake is great to have made up in advance – you can throw it in the oven when you have a shorter, harder session to do on the bike

Life's too short to make your own gnocchi, especially when there are some really good readymade versions available. It's a welcome change from the starchy staples of rice, pasta and potatoes too. There's a little bit of a faff involved in putting this together, but it is really easy and you can still knock it up in less than 30 minutes. The key to success is don't over-cook the gnocchi and veg.

Serves 2 as a main meal with a portion left over for lunch

1 head of broccoli, trimmed and chopped

500 g (1 lb 2 oz) gluten-free gnocchi

3 teaspoons olive oil

1 large bag (500 g / 1 lb 2 oz) baby spinach leaves

sea salt and freshly ground black pepper

500 g (1 lb 2 oz) chicken mini breast fillets

2 garlic cloves, peeled and roughly chopped

100 g (3 ½ oz) chestnut mushrooms, peeled and chopped

100 ml (½ cup) single cream

100 g (3 ½ oz) low-fat cream cheese

about 2 tablespoons chopped fresh tarragon

3 tablespoons grated strong hard cheese, such as Parmesan or Pecorino

1 bunch of spring onions, trimmed and sliced, to serve

Nutrition per serving:
Calories 827 | Total carbohydrate 72 g | Sugars 10 g
Fat 30 g | Protein 71 g | Sodium 585 mg

1. First, preheat the oven to 190°C/375°F/Gas 5. Now, put a large pan of boiling salted water on (pre-boil the water in a kettle) and then place a sauté pan on another ring on low to warm through. If you do these two things at once, this recipe is really quick.

2. Add the broccoli to the boiling water, reduce the heat and simmer for 3 minutes max. Strain off through a sieve or colander and set aside, leaving the cooking water in the pan. Bring the cooking liquid back to the boil and cook the gnocchi for 60 seconds max, strain off and set aside.

3. Heat 1 teaspoon of the olive oil in the sauté pan and fry the spinach over a high heat for 60 seconds. Season well and press out any excess liquid with a wooden spoon; set aside.

4. Add a teaspoon of olive oil to the sauté pan and fry the chicken on both sides with the garlic for 5–6 minutes. Season well and set aside. Finally, sauté the mushrooms in the same pan in the remaining oil for 2–3 minutes over a high heat and set aside.

5. Mix together the cream and cream cheese in a bowl and season well. Stir the tarragon into the cream mix.

6. Line the base of a casserole dish with the spinach, then layer with gnocchi, then broccoli, chicken and mushrooms. Pour over the cream mix, season and sprinkle with cheese. Bake in the centre of the oven for 20–30 minutes. Serve sprinkled with chopped spring onions to finish off.

Grilled salmon with fresh asparagus, pea, mint and basil risotto

A lovely, fresh-tasting way of serving good-quality starchy carbs

The risotto base works with so many different forms of protein: try it with grilled lamb chops or even chunks of feta cheese as a vegetarian option. If asparagus is unavailable, broccoli works just as well.

Serves 2 with a good portion of risotto left over for lunch

25 g (1 oz) unsalted butter

1 onion, peeled and chopped

200 g (7 oz) Arborio (risotto) rice

600 ml (2 ½ cups) vegetable stock (good-quality stock cubes or shop-bought stock)

250 g (9 oz) defrosted frozen peas for the purée and 75 g (3 oz) to stir through the rice

1 tablespoon extra virgin olive oil

sea salt and freshly ground black pepper

1 teaspoon olive oil

2 x 125 g (4 oz) fresh salmon fillets

juice of half a lemon

small bunch of fresh mint, chopped

6 basil leaves, torn

12 medium spears fresh cooked asparagus

Nutrition per serving:

Calories 968 | Total carbohydrate 111 g | Sugars 14 g
Fat 37 g | Protein 51 g | Sodium 349 mg

1. Preheat a large saucepan over a low heat. Melt the butter and add the chopped onion. Fry gently for 2–3 minutes until softened. Stir in the rice and cook over a medium heat for a further 2 minutes – no colour on the rice, please.

2. The next stage is to add the stock and simmer for 16–18 minutes until all the liquid has been absorbed and the rice is softened. Note: we want the rice mix to be quite dry so keep stirring every so often as it cooks.

3. While the rice is cooking, in a food processor blend 250 g (9 oz) of the peas with the extra virgin olive oil, season and set aside. Note: we still want some texture in the peas so only blend until slightly crushed.

4. Preheat the grill to a medium heat. Meanwhile, use a pastry brush to brush the salmon fillets with the olive oil and place under the grill for 6–7 minutes. Finish with lemon juice.

5. Once the risotto rice is cooked, stir in the puréed pea mix. Reheat the risotto mix and the asparagus separately. Add the remaining 75 g (3 oz) peas, fresh mint and basil to the risotto. Adjust the seasoning, transfer to plates and serve with the grilled salmon and asparagus spears.

Big Mike's Moroccan tagine

A firm favourite with my cycling friends, this is comfort food that is high in protein, low in fat and extremely flavoursome

Big Mike is an old friend and the best cook I know who is not a chef. This one-pot dish is adapted from his classic, which I can't really improve. The key here is adding the fresh herbs at the last minute. If you can't find a Moroccan spice mix, Ras-el-Hanout is widely available in supermarkets and will work just as well. This is a great meal to batch-cook or have as leftovers for lunch. Serve with steamed couscous for a truly authentic Moroccan meal.

Serves 4

2 tablespoons olive oil

500 g (1 lb 2 oz) skinless chicken breast, diced

3 teaspoons Moroccan spice mix

1 tablespoon 'lazy' chopped garlic

3 mixed peppers, deseeded and diced

1 large white onion, peeled and diced

1 tin (215 g / 7 ½ oz drained weight) chickpeas, strained

1 tin (400 g / 14 oz) chopped plum tomatoes

400 ml (1 ½ cups) chicken stock (good-quality stock cubes or shop-bought stock)

steamed couscous (cook according to the packet directions), to serve

sea salt and freshly ground black pepper

1 bunch each, finely chopped, fresh mint, parsley and coriander

75 g (3 oz) chopped dried apricots and 25 g (1 oz) flaked almonds, to finish

Nutrition per serving:
Calories 402 | Total carbohydrate 28 g | Sugars 17 g
Fat 15 g | Protein 37 g | Sodium 647 mg

1. Preheat a large non-stick saucepan. Heat the olive oil and gently sauté the diced chicken, turning, for 3–4 minutes until lightly coloured.

2. Stir in the Moroccan spice mix and cook for a further 2 minutes before adding the garlic, peppers and onion. Cook over a medium heat for a further 2 minutes.

3. The next stage is to add the chickpeas, plum tomatoes and chicken stock. Bring to the boil and simmer gently, stirring occasionally, for 30–40 minutes. While the tagine is cooking, make the couscous according to the directions on the packet.

4. Adjust the seasoning for the tagine and at the last minute remove from the heat and stir in the fresh herbs. Divide the couscous between plates and top with tagine. Serve sprinkled with apricots and almonds.

Variations

Lamb shoulder would be also be great in this dish, as opposed to chicken. Use 500 g (1 lb 2 oz) of diced lamb shoulder. If you use lamb, increase the cooking time to 90 minutes and increase the amount of stock by 50 per cent. If you are feeling flash, finish with a sprinkling of pomegranate seeds.

Vegan Thai red curry with coconut, red lentils and coriander

A cracking way of eating a hearty meal with minimal cost! Protein comes from the lentils and the recipe is vegan-friendly too

Meat such as chicken or turkey can easily be incorporated into this meal by adding at the same time as the veg, but in all honesty, you won't miss it. You can make the base up in advance, just be sure to add the coriander at the last minute to retain the freshness of its flavour.

Serves 4

2 tablespoons olive oil

550 g (1 lb 3 oz) butternut squash, diced

2 large carrots, trimmed and diced

2 large sweet potatoes, peeled and diced

1 white onion, peeled and chopped

2 red peppers, deseeded and sliced

1–2 teaspoons Thai red curry paste

250 g (9 oz) red lentils

400 ml (1 ½ cups) coconut milk

400 ml (1 ½ cups) vegetable stock (good-quality stock cubes or shop-bought stock)

basmati rice or rice noodles (cook according to the packet directions), to serve

juice of 1 lime

1 teaspoon soy sauce

1 bunch of fresh coriander, chopped

75 g (3 oz) salted peanuts

Nutrition per serving:

Calories 568 | Total carbohydrate 58 g | Sugars 15 g
Fat 32 g | Protein 15 g | Sodium 609 mg

1. Heat the olive oil in a large saucepan. Add all the vegetables and cook over a medium heat for 5–6 minutes until the veg has a little colour.

2. Add the Thai curry paste and cook for a further 2 minutes. Now, I have given you an option of 1–2 teaspoons. This depends on how hot you like your curry and also how hot the individual paste is – it's easier to add more than take it out!

3. Next, stir in the lentils, coconut milk and stock. Simmer for 25–30 minutes over a low to medium heat, or you can even cook it on a medium heat in a slow cooker. If cooking in a pan, make sure you stir the mix every now and then to ensure the lentils don't catch.

4. While the curry is cooking, prepare the rice or rice noodles. Once the lentils have softened and the veg is cooked, season with the lime juice and soy sauce. Divide the rice or rice noodles between your plates, top with the curry and then add the chopped coriander at the last minute. Serve sprinkled with peanuts.

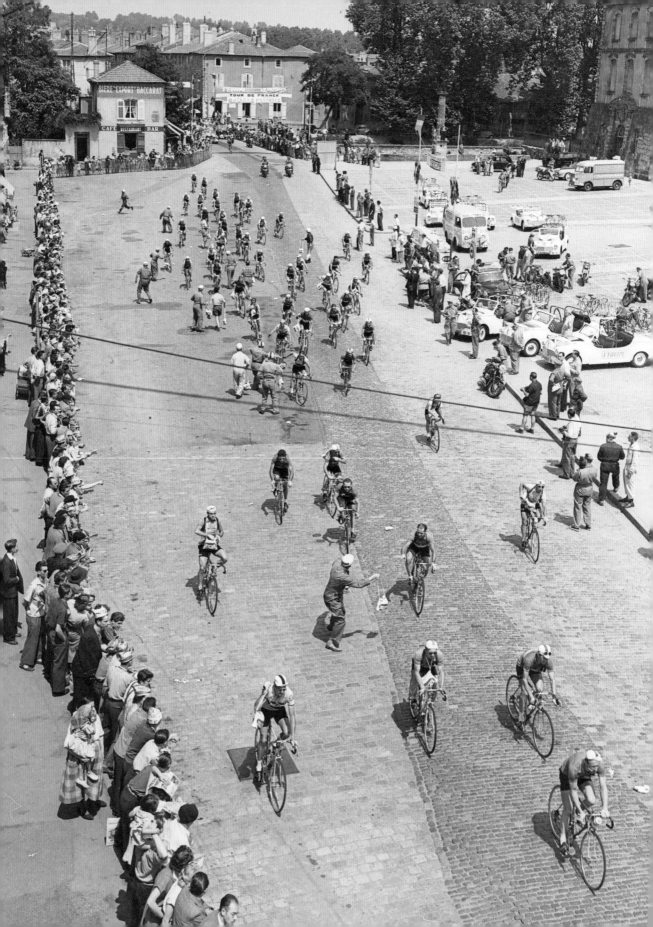

High-Performance Diet on a Budget

When it comes to meals and snacks, high performance doesn't have to mean high expenditure. A well-planned trip to the supermarket can give you all you need for a nutritious and balanced diet.

You may not be able to afford skinsuits, £10k bikes or access to wind tunnels, but you can replicate a professional's diet on a reasonable budget, because it's based on simple, natural food. All the food necessary to race and recover is available from your local supermarket and so it's really quite easy to eat to the same nutritional standard as the pro peloton.

Riders take on supplies at a food station during the 1955 Tour de France. It is possible to replicate a professional's diet on a reasonable budget. All the food necessary to race and recover is available from your local supermarket.

Essential Budget Ingredients

- Rice – dry or pre-cooked
- Oats – supermarket value 1 kg bags
- Pasta – supermarket raw pasta
- Tinned tomatoes
- Tinned sweetcorn
- Tinned pulses
- Tinned fish
- Peanut butter
- Frozen peas and other vegetables
- Yoghurts.

Ingredients Worth the Extra Expense

- Nuts and berries
- Fresh meat and fish
- Organic eggs
- Organic milk
- Olive oil (regular and extra virgin)
- Fresh herbs
- Dijon mustard – a great companion to oily fish, especially if you don't like fish!
- Good-quality stock cubes.

Whatever your budget, your shopping basket should contain fresh fruit, vegetables, fish and meat, pulses (dried lentils and tinned beans), pasta and bread. You don't need to compromise on fuel. The choice of meat, fish or vegetables depends on what you like and what you can afford. It isn't essential to have meat at every single meal – many elite cyclists have two or three vegetarian or vegan days a week – and you don't have to choose expensive fish, because coley or hake deliver the same benefits as a really expensive piece of turbot or sea bass.

Don't feel you have to buy organic fruit and veg – the nutritional benefits are generally not worth the expense – and don't shun own-brand, value-label goods, because the food inside is pretty similar. Just be alert. In your attempts to keep spending and cooking time to a minimum you might be tempted by a cheap ready meal or other heavily processed pre-packaged foodstuffs, but this will be a false economy, because they're stripped of virtually all nutrients and packed with additives, preservatives, sugar or salt.

Much of what you need is simple and cheap. Porridge oats can form the basis of a varied, easily digestible and carb-packed breakfast. Eggs really are a cyclist's best friend, because they're an inexpensive source of high-quality protein, versatile and easy to cook. Turkey is not just for Christmas – it's excellent lean protein and usually cheaper than chicken. And tins of oily fish? What a godsend! When I get in from a hard ride, what I really love is sardines on toast. It's about as complete a post-ride meal as you can make, and it's cooked and eaten in minutes. Tuna, avocado and rice make for a superb recovery supper too – if you're too exhausted to cook the rice, just use pre-cooked pouches.

It's not what's in your wallet that will prevent you following a high-performance diet: the key is the ability to plan and make appetising food that you're going to want to eat. Eating to a training plan will ensure you align input with output. Where possible, cook in bulk and freeze in individual meal-sized containers. It'll save time and money, ensure that you have food ready when you need it and allow you to control portion sizes.

A decent blender should also be up there alongside that new GPS on your wish list. It unlocks the power of the smoothie, a fantastic source of protein, antioxidants and vitamins, which, better still, can be packed full of cheap ingredients. Superfoods don't have to be exotic – chuck in kale, pre-cooked beetroot, frozen berries and whatever fresh fruit is available, and blend into a great breakfast, energy supplement or recovery meal.

Meanwhile, on the road, although energy bars have their uses, why not spend a little of your recovery time making the bike snacks in this book? (*See also* p. 154.) They're a lot tastier than anything you'll buy at the supermarket and a fraction of the price. And for all your supplements and gels, I take a simple nut butter and jam roll on a long ride, because it's a near-perfect ratio of calories to proteins and carbs.

This will all make for super-efficient shopping, which is great, because it's worth saving every penny for some non-budget essentials. Only ever use organic milk and try mixing it with soya, brown rice or almond milk to aid digestion – you'll see it on the pro teams' breakfast tables. Organic eggs pack more nutritional value into their yolks and are worth the higher price. And be fussy about bread. Despite the attractively low price, sliced loaves and products from in-store bakeries contain numerous additives and should be avoided. If you can, find a freshly made organic loaf or, better still, leave the supermarket and visit a local bakery or farmers' market.

Must-follow Rules

- Plan your meals in advance and shop accordingly.
- Budget for all nutrient groups – skipping meat or fish is a false economy and good value options are available.
- Always check for additives and avoid heavily processed foods.
- Have recovery food ready to hand – the worst shopping decisions are made when you're hungry and tired!
- Allow yourself a treat every now and then – don't allow eating to become a joyless experience. Remember also that life sometimes gets in the way – it's essential to enjoy a special family meal out, Christmas dinner or celebration without feeling guilty.

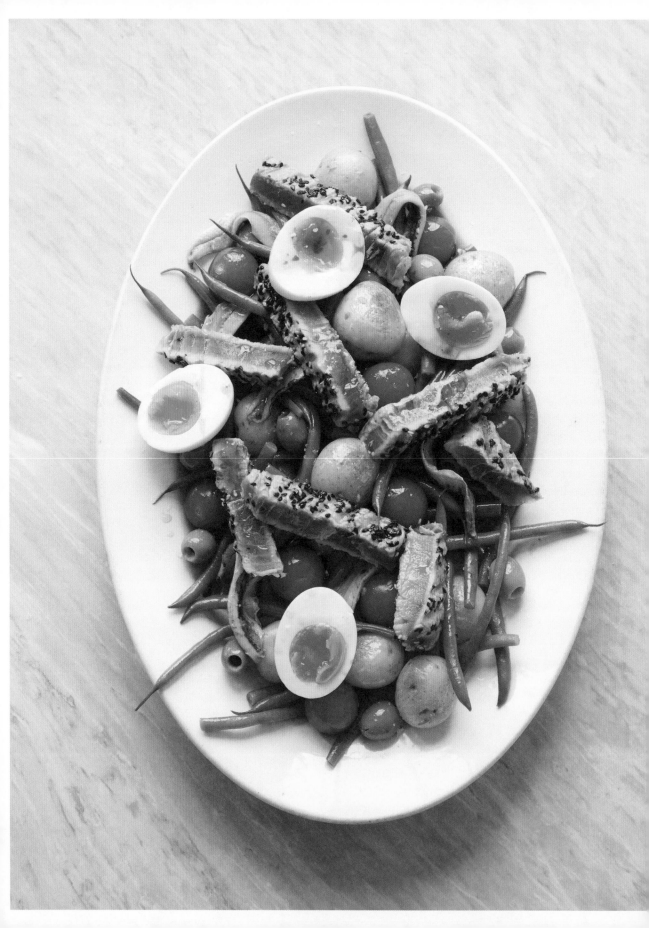

Sesame and soy tuna niçoise

Fresh tuna provides an excellent source of vitamin D, which can boost aerobic capacity and shorten recovery time

The key to this dish is finding a nice chunk of tuna. This is relatively easy to do and it's a far superior product to the tinned variety, not that I'm totally against tinned fish. Also, look for *boquerones* – the best white anchovies you can find, pickled in vinegar and olive oil. I also like to add a little bit of Asia to this dish by using some soy sauce to deglaze the tuna and in the dressing too.

Serves 2

300 g (11 oz) green beans

sea salt

12 new potatoes (6 per person)

2 teaspoons unsalted butter

1 teaspoon olive oil

1 teaspoon black sesame seeds

1 teaspoon white sesame seeds

2 x tuna steaks (150–170 g / 5–6 oz per person)

1 tablespoon soy sauce

10 cherry vine tomatoes

16 green olives

12 *boquerones* (white anchovies)

2–3 boiled eggs

Dressing

30 ml (1 ½ tablespoons) soy sauce

20 ml (1 tablespoon) white wine vinegar

50 ml (3 tablespoons) water

75 ml (4 ½ tablespoons) olive oil

25 ml (1 ½ tablespoons) sesame oil

1 tablespoon black sesame seeds

1 tablespoon white sesame seeds

1. Start the process by cooking the green beans in boiling salted water for 3–4 minutes, then drain and set aside. Also, pre-cook the new potatoes: to finish, slice in half and then sauté in butter over a medium heat for 6–8 minutes.

2. To cook the tuna, preheat a grill pan and get it really hot. Add the olive oil to the pan, sprinkle the sesame seeds over both sides of the tuna and then sear for no more than 20 seconds on each side. At the last minute add the soy sauce to glaze the tuna, then remove from the pan to stop the cooking process.

3. Make your dressing by mixing all the ingredients together (shake in a jar or whisk in a bowl). This dressing will keep for up to a month stored in an airtight jar in the fridge.

4. Assembling the dish could not be easier: arrange all the vegetables and the tomatoes on a plate. Add the olives and boquerones. Slice the tuna and arrange on top, halve the boiled eggs and place these on top as well, then spoon over some of the dressing – banging!

Nutrition per serving:

Calories 618 | Total carbohydrate 35 g | Sugars 7 g | Fat 27 g
Protein 61 g | Sodium 418 mg

Venison sausages with roasted beetroot and red onion

Venison is the ultimate red meat as it is high in iron and lower in fat than other types of red meat

This roasted veg number would also work well with carrots, butternut squash, sweet potato and Jerusalem artichokes.

Serves 2

350 g (12 oz) raw peeled beetroot

1 medium celeriac

4 medium red onions

2 tablespoons olive oil (extra for brushing)

sea salt and freshly ground black pepper

a few sprigs of fresh rosemary and thyme

1 tablespoon balsamic vinegar

1 x 300 g (11 oz) pack venison sausages

Nutrition per serving:
Calories 627 | Total carbohydrate 44 g | Sugars 18 g
Fat 30 g | Protein 29 g | Sodium 1104 mg

1. Preheat the oven to 190°C/375°F/Gas 5. Slice the beetroot and celeriac into similar sized chunks and peel and cut the onions into quarters. Place all the veg in the casserole pan with the olive oil, season well and place in the centre of the oven for 20 minutes, stirring halfway through.

2. Add the herbs and the balsamic vinegar to the mix. Stir once and return to the oven for a further 10 minutes.

3. While the veg are cooking, it's time to cook the venison sausages. Preheat the grill to medium heat. Use a pastry brush to brush the sausages with a little oil and then grill for 8–10 minutes, turning a couple of times. Arrange the roasted veg on plates and serve with the grilled sausages.

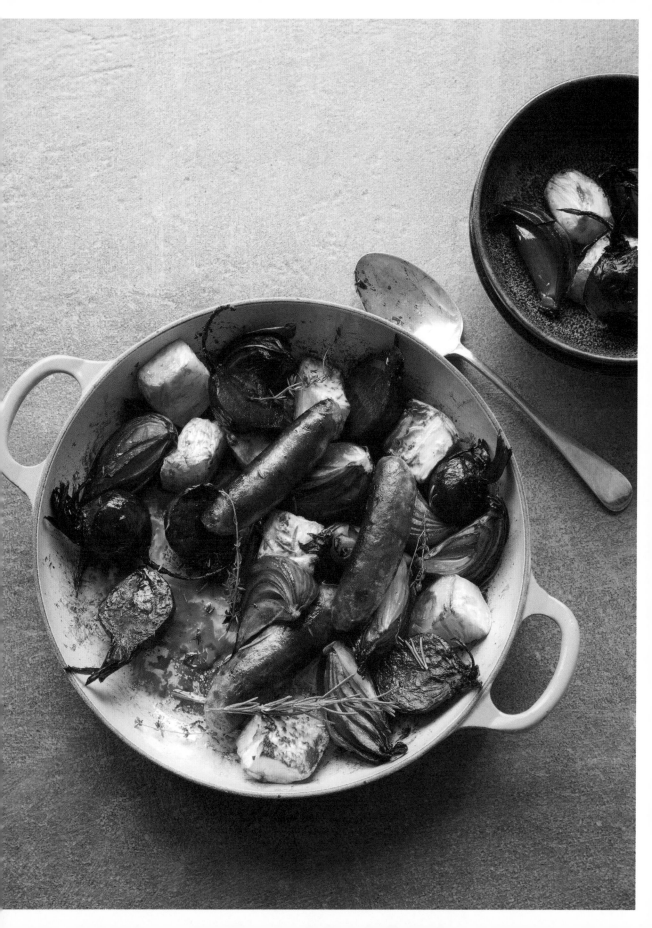

Chicken and avocado Caesar salad

Avocados are a great source of healthy fats. They're also full of vitamins, minerals and antioxidants (compounds that help repair muscle damage)

A good Caesar salad is hard to beat! Here I have adapted it slightly with the addition of some grilled chicken and avocado, so it's more of a proper meal than just a plate of lettuce.

Serves 2

8 chicken mini fillets (4 per person – 180 g / 6 oz)

2 teaspoons olive oil

sea salt and freshly ground black pepper

2 small slices of bread, diced and cut into croutons

2 heads of romaine lettuce

1 large avocado, peeled, pitted and diced

2 tablespoons low-fat Caesar dressing

10 *boquerones* (white anchovies)

2 tablespoons finely grated Parmesan

1. Preheat the grill to medium/high heat. Using a pastry brush, brush the chicken fillets with half the olive oil. Season and grill for 8 minutes.

2. While the chicken is grilling, toss the croutons in a bowl with the remaining oil. Season well and fry in a non-stick pan for 5–6 minutes over a low to medium heat until golden brown.

3. Shred the lettuce into a serving bowl. Mix with the chopped avocado and the dressing. Arrange the anchovies, croutons and grilled chicken on top, sprinkle with Parmesan and get stuck in!

Nutrition per serving:

Calories 623 | Total carbohydrate 27 g | Sugars 4 g | Fat 25 g
Protein 74 g | Sodium 445 mg

Cod fillet with pumpkin seed and pine nut tabbouleh

This meal can be cooked really quickly and provides a fantastic mix of protein and carbohydrates

Couscous is a really simple grain to work with. Just add boiling water and leave it for 10 minutes and, boom, you are there! You can choose any delicate white fish to serve with the couscous – as always, the freshness of the fish is more important than the actual variety.

Serves 2

150 g (5 oz) couscous

500 ml (2 cups) water

50 ml (3 tablespoons) lemon juice
(extra to serve)

zest of 1 lemon

50 ml (3 tablespoons) olive oil (extra for brushing)

1 tablespoon crushed coriander seeds

2 tablespoons pumpkin seeds

2 tablespoons pine nuts

1 small bunch coriander, finely chopped

sea salt and freshly ground black pepper

2 x cod fillets (150–200 g / 5–7 oz
per person)

large green salad, to serve

1. Start by cooking the couscous. Place it in a large heatproof bowl, boil a kettle and add 500 ml (2 cups) of boiling water to the grains. Stir and cover for 10 minutes, then break up the grains with a fork. Stir in the lemon juice, zest and olive oil.

2. Toast off your seeds and pine nuts in a dry pan, shaking the pan every so often. Keep an eye on them as they will burn the second your back is turned. Add to the lemon couscous. Stir in the coriander and adjust the seasoning. The mix is served at room temperature.

3. Preheat the grill to medium heat. Using a pastry brush, brush the cod fillets with a touch of olive oil. Grill for 6–7 minutes, season and add a touch of lemon juice. Serve with the couscous and a large green salad.

Nutrition per serving:
Calories 828 | Total carbohydrate 63 g | Sugars 1 g
Fat 44 g | Protein 47 g | Sodium 12 mg

Avocado coleslaw with greens and cold smoked salmon

All the beautiful richness and crunch of a traditional coleslaw combined with the benefit of the good fats from the avocado

This lovely fresh dish was borne out of necessity. I came in from a ride and there wasn't much in the fridge apart from a load of old veg and a couple of overripe avocados! We don't tend to think of coleslaw as a healthy food, but I have had a play about and made a rich creamy dressing for sliced veg using avocado. This recipe would also work really well with smoked or grilled chicken. You can use any type of raw green veg – spring cabbage, watercress, Savoy cabbage, spinach, kale, courgetti, etc., but you need a good percentage of onion to ensure you have the acidity and crunch of a traditional coleslaw.

Serves 4

¼ of a Savoy cabbage

½ of a spring green cabbage

1 large white onion, peeled

1 head of pak choi

1 small bunch of spring onions, trimmed

200 g (7 oz) avocado flesh

50 ml (3 tablespoons) extra virgin olive oil

50 ml (3 tablespoons) lemon juice

150 g (5 oz) low-fat crème fraîche

sea salt and ground black pepper

200 g (7 oz) cold smoked salmon

50 g (2 oz) sunflower seeds

50 g (2 oz) pumpkin seeds, toasted

1. Finely slice up the all the vegetables and set aside.

2. Now, make the avocado 'mayonnaise' by placing the avocado flesh with the olive oil, lemon juice, crème fraîche and a good pinch of sea salt in the bowl of a food processor. Blend until a smooth silky texture has been achieved. Correct the seasoning, then transfer to a large serving bowl and mix in the sliced vegetables.

3. Finely slice your smoked salmon and serve with the avocado slaw, topped with the sunflower and pumpkin seeds.

Nutrition per serving:
Calories 552 | Total carbohydrate 18 g | Sugars 8 g | Fat 38 g
Protein 22 g | Sodium 24 mg

Grilled sea trout with peas, bacon and lettuce

Trout is a healthy and sustainable fish with a relatively low total fat and saturated fat content compared to other oily fish

Cooked lettuce… bear with me here. A take on a French classic, *Petits Pois à la Française*, this is a lovely light fish dish served with smoked bacon, cooked lettuce and peas – all done last minute. It doesn't keep well or reheat, so please do everything just before you want to eat. If you are having a hungry day, serve with some boiled new potatoes.

Serves 2

1 tablespoon olive oil (extra for brushing)

150 g (5 oz) good-quality smoked bacon, chopped

1 medium onion, peeled and finely sliced

2 sea trout fillets (150 g / 5 oz each)

sea salt and freshly ground black pepper

4 Little Gem lettuces

300 g (11 oz) frozen peas, defrosted

squeeze of lemon juice

1. Heat the olive oil in a pan set over a medium heat. Fry the bacon and onion for 4 minutes – you don't want it to colour, just to cook through.

2. Preheat the grill to a high heat. Using a pastry brush, brush the sea trout with a little olive oil, season and place under the grill for 4–5 minutes, turning halfway through the cooking time.

3. Meanwhile, slice the lettuce into quarters and add to the bacon and onion mix; cook over a low heat for a further 2–3 minutes. Add the defrosted peas and cook for a further 2 minutes. Add a decent squeeze of lemon juice and adjust the seasoning. Transfer to plates and serve topped with the trout.

Nutrition per serving:
Calories 618 | Total carbohydrate 31 g | Sugars 12 g
Fat 28 g | Protein 63 g | Sodium 3235 mg

Smoked mackerel with watercress salad, beetroot and grainy mustard new potatoes

Combined with the good fats from the mackerel, the addition of watercress makes this dish highly nutritious

One of my favourite fish to work with, mackerel is really good value and widely available. This is a very simple dish and the only cooking you need to do is boiling some new potatoes. Watercress is high in antioxidants, with a slightly bitter, peppery flavour. It's one of the boldest salad leaves out there. It grows wild in my adopted home county of Hampshire and riding past the watercress beds has provided the inspiration for many of my recipes.

Serves 2

12 new potatoes

sea salt and freshly ground black pepper

1 tablespoon grainy mustard

1 teaspoon white wine vinegar

1 teaspoon extra virgin olive oil

200 g (7 oz) smoked mackerel fillets

100 g (3 ½ oz) cooked beetroot

1 bunch of fresh watercress

Nutrition per serving:
Calories 416 | Total carbohydrate 28 g | Sugars 5 g
Fat 23 g | Protein 21 g | Sodium 323 mg

1. Slice the potatoes in half and simmer in boiling salted water for 10–12 minutes until cooked. Strain off the water, transfer the potatoes to a bowl and immediately combine with the mustard, vinegar and olive oil. Adjust the seasoning and set aside. This is all your physical cooking done!

2. Remove the skin from the mackerel and roughly flake up the fish, then dice the beetroot and pick your watercress leaves. Arrange all the ingredients together on a plate and serve at once.

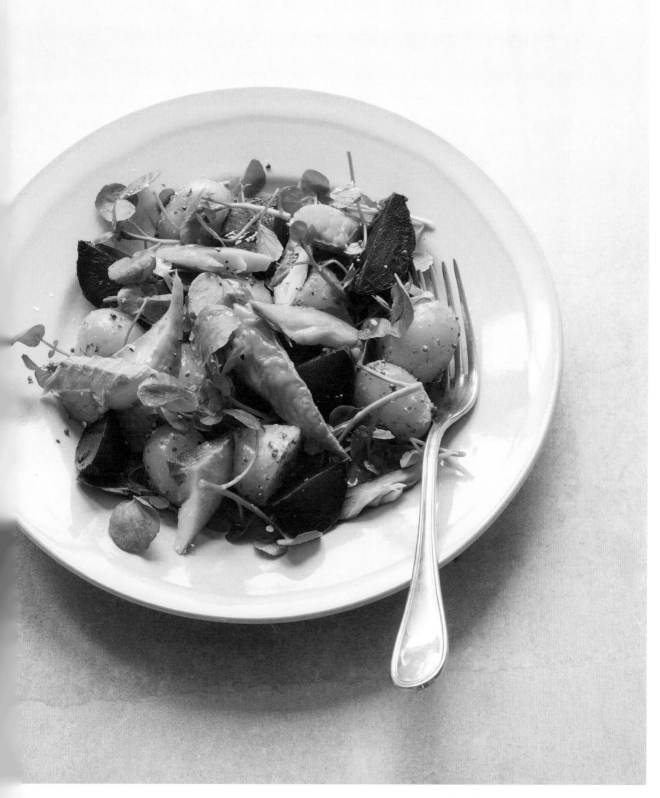

Greek yoghurt with avocado, green pepper, coriander and mango

A light and refreshing lunchtime dish, full of goodness and ideal for a rest day or anytime you have a reduced training load

Good levels of protein and good fats, lovely textures and no actual cooking required – simple!

Serves 2

300 g (11 oz) full-fat Greek yoghurt

2 medium avocado, peeled, pitted
and chopped

2 tablespoons chopped fresh mango

1 teaspoon finely diced green chilli

1 tablespoon diced green pepper

1 tablespoon chopped fresh coriander

2 teaspoons extra virgin olive oil

a squeeze of fresh lime juice

a good pinch of sea salt

a good handful (30 g / 1 ½ oz) of corn
tortilla chips

Nutrition per serving:
Calories 611 | Total carbohydrate 48 g | Sugars 23 g
Fat 44 g | Protein 12 g | Sodium 278 mg

1. So very simple: into a bowl with the Greek yoghurt, top with the remaining ingredients and away you go!

Grilled halibut with pickled fennel, dill and orange

Orange zest actually contains higher amounts of certain nutrients than the flesh, so this recipe gives an extra boost as well as a big punch of flavour.

Orange and fennel are a lovely combination to complement fish. Fennel is a very under-appreciated veg – most people don't know what to do with it. The citrus and aniseed flavours here work really well together. You could serve almost any type of fish with this flavour combination – cod would be particularly good.

Serves 2

2 heads of fennel

1 large red onion, trimmed and peeled

1 head of chicory

2 medium oranges

1 teaspoon white wine vinegar

2 tablespoons extra virgin olive oil (extra for grilling)

2 halibut fillets (about 150–200 g / 5–7 oz per person)

sea salt and ground black pepper

1 small bunch of dill

1 teaspoon fennel seeds

Nutrition per serving:

Calories 498 | Total carbohydrate 41 g | Sugars 25 g
Fat 20 g | Protein 41 g | Sodium 217 mg

1. Start by slicing the fennel, red onion and chicory very finely. Mix together in a heatproof bowl and set aside.

2. Grate the zest from the oranges and place in a small saucepan. Segment one of the oranges and put the segments to one side. Squeeze the juice from the trim and the remaining orange and place in the saucepan with the white wine vinegar and the orange zest. Set over a medium heat and boil the juice for 3 minutes.

3. Add the extra virgin olive oil and simmer for a further 60 seconds, then pour the hot liquid onto the sliced veg. Leave to marinate for 15 minutes: the acid in the orange and vinegar will break down the fennel mix.

4. Meanwhile, preheat the grill to a high heat. Brush the halibut fillets with a touch of olive oil and season well. Grill for 4–5 minutes.

5. To finish the dish off, chop the dill and mix with the orange segments, pickled veg and the fennel seeds. Arrange on plates with the halibut fillets and serve at once.

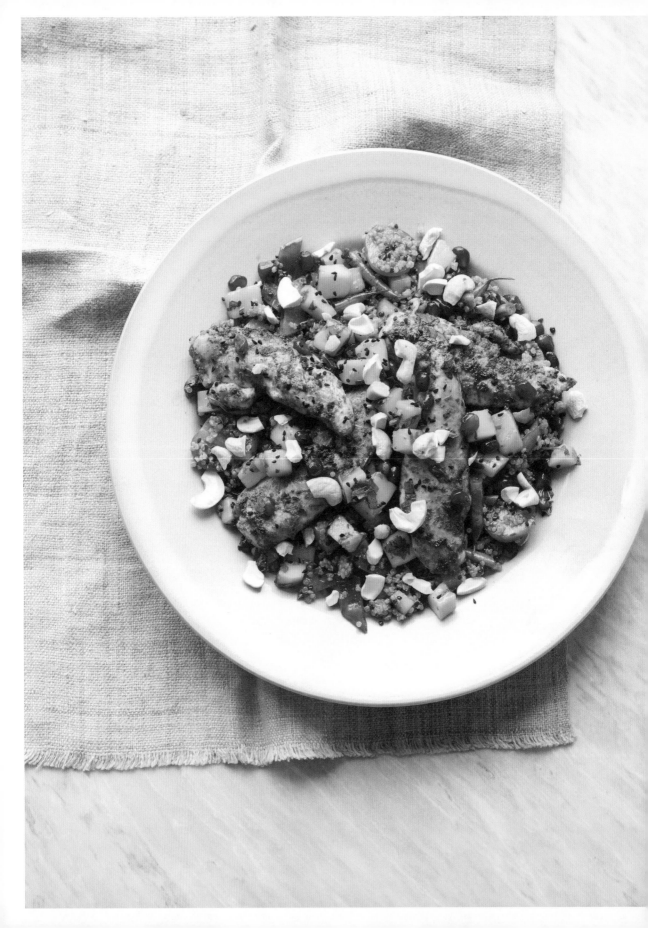

BBQ spiced chicken with quinoa, mango and pomegranate salsa

Quinoa is widely regarded as the ultimate grain. This is perfect as a recovery meal or as a lunchtime meal ahead of an evening ride

This dish delivers decent levels of protein and carbs, with interesting textures and flavour combinations. The balance of sweet and salty works so well, while the raw veg mixed with the quinoa livens up a pretty bland base grain. The beauty of this meal is that it can easily be put together in no time at all and can be made up in advance. There is not a cyclist I advise who hasn't had this meal and loved it.

Serves 2

250 g (9 oz) pre-cooked quinoa

100 g (3 ½ oz) diced cucumber or courgettes

2 tomatoes, chopped

50 g (2 oz) green beans, chopped

50 g (2 oz) mangetouts, chopped

sea salt and freshly ground black pepper

8–10 chicken mini fillets (about 150 g / 5 oz chicken per person)

2 tablespoons cajun or BBQ spice mix

2 teaspoons olive oil

25 g (1 oz) chopped cashews

a pinch of black onion seeds

a handful of baby spinach

Salsa

1 medium ripe mango, peeled and pitted

1 pack of pre-prepared pomegranate seeds (80 g / 3 oz)

small bunch of fresh mint

small bunch of fresh coriander

Dressing

1 tablespoon Thai fish sauce

1 tablespoon soy sauce

1 tablespoon sweet chilli sauce

1 tablespoon extra virgin olive oil

1. To make the dressing, whisk the Thai fish sauce, soy sauce, sweet chilli sauce and extra virgin olive oil in a large bowl. Combine the cooked quinoa with half the dressing. Add the diced cucumber or courgettes, tomatoes, green beans and mangetouts. Adjust the seasoning and set aside.

2. Make the salsa by first dicing the mango. Transfer to a bowl and mix with the pomegranate seeds, mint and coriander. Stir into the remaining dressing.

3. To make the spiced chicken, dice the chicken and marinate with the cajun or BBQ spice mix for 5 minutes (allow 1 teaspoon of mild spice and 1 teaspoon of olive oil per 150 g / 5 oz chicken). Grill under a medium heat or pan-fry for 4–5 minutes until the chicken is cooked through.

4. Arrange the quinoa salad, salsa and spiced chicken on plates. Sprinkle over the chopped cashews and black onion seeds. Serve warm or at room temperature with the baby spinach leaves for the perfect balanced meal.

Nutrition per serving:

Calories 887 | Total carbohydrate 97 g | Sugars 42 g | Fat 28 g
Protein 65 g | Sodium 590 mg

Eggs

Eggs are the cyclist's best friend. Someone should wrap them up and sell them in bike shops next to the gels and protein powders. They'd make a fortune. These little gems are a complete protein package and more besides.

If you need convincing, here's the nutritional headlines: eggs contain all 20 amino acids required by the body; they fill you up effectively; and they are one of the few foods containing natural vitamin D as well as other essential minerals and vitamins. In cyclists' terms, a couple of scrambled eggs are the perfect addition to carbohydrates to provide energy for a ride, and a three-egg omelette provides the ideal building blocks for muscle repair after a long ride.

Fortunately, science did a U-turn on eggs some years back. While once we were advised not to eat eggs daily because of cholesterol and fat concerns, advice from health bodies such as the NHS in the UK has dismissed such theories. Two or three small eggs a day should cause no problems for a healthy adult.

That's just as well, as they are such a quick and easy option for breakfast, lunch and dinner. Obviously you can make omelettes and pancakes, or scramble and poach them, but you could also fry them up with cooked rice for a power snack or take a boiled egg or an egg muffin with you for an on-the-bike boost.

One note, whenever possible, is to opt for organic free-range eggs. Whatever your ethical views on caged birds never seeing sunlight, their eggs will simply never be the same quality as those from birds that roam freely and eat insects and plants. The nutritional values of free-range eggs are much denser and the rich yolks much more flavoursome.

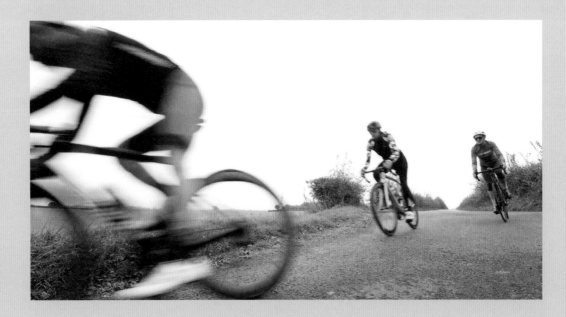

Poached eggs, smoked salmon, avocado and pumpkin seed mash

A great post-ride lunch or a lighter dinner, this has pretty much everything you need in one balanced meal

Poached eggs with avocado on toast is one dish that is on the menu of pretty much every health-conscious restaurant. It hits all the food groups: carbs, good fats and protein. This is my take on it. Here I have added pumpkin seeds (which I love) and also smoked salmon to turn it into a proper meal. Mastering a decent poached egg is an essential life skill, so follow the steps below. The freshness of the egg determines the success of this dish… oh, and a little bit of cheffing technique!

Serves 2

1 teaspoon sea salt

50 ml (3 tablespoons) white vinegar

1 large ripe avocado, peeled and pitted

1 tablespoon extra virgin olive oil

1 teaspoon lemon juice (or white wine vinegar)

30 g (1 ½ oz) pumpkin seeds

sea salt and freshly ground black pepper

4 large free-range eggs

4 slices of good-quality bread for toasting

100 g (3 ½ oz) sliced cold smoked salmon

Nutrition per serving:

Calories 755 | Total carbohydrate 51 g | Sugars 3 g | Fat 46 g
Protein 38 g | Sodium 158 mg

1. Start by placing a shallow-sided pan of boiling water on to boil – the water needs to about 6 cm (2.5 inch) deep. Add the sea salt and the white vinegar to the water and simmer gently.

2. The next thing to do is to make your mashed avocado: place the ripe avocado flesh in a bowl and crush with a fork. Stir in the olive oil, lemon juice and pumpkin seeds. Season well and set aside.

3. Now, crack the eggs into a small bowl, then gently whisk the boiling water with a fork to form a whirlpool effect. Carefully pour the eggs into the centre of the whirlpool. Simmer gently for 3–4 minutes until the whites have firmed up. Aim to keep the yolks nice and runny; this might take you a few attempts to get it right, so keep practising whenever you make this dish.

4. While the eggs are cooking, toast the bread and arrange on plates. Top with smoked salmon and a dollop of avocado mash. Once cooked, remove the eggs from the water with a slotted spoon. Place on top of the smoked salmon/avocado mash and serve sprinkled with a little freshly ground black pepper.

Dutch omelette, roasted Brussels sprouts with smoked ham and sage

High in protein, this is great for post-ride refuelling after a short, hard session

Dutch omelette? There I was in a restaurant in Holland, having been racing. I was feeling pretty tired and had little appetite, but when I saw the most random dish ever – Brussels sprout omelette – I thought I'd try it. It was horrendous, with over-cooked sprouts that were cold in the middle. But when I came home, I adapted the dish as I love Brussels sprouts, which are high in fibre and vitamin C. When you sauté them, you get a really great flavour and texture. This omelette also works really well with sautéed broccoli. For a veggie option, omit the ham.

Serves 1

100 g (3 ½ oz) raw Brussels sprouts

1 tablespoon olive oil

sea salt and ground black pepper

1 knob of unsalted butter

3–4 leaves fresh sage, chopped

3 large free-range eggs

1 tablespoon milk

50 g (2 oz) smoked ham

Large green salad, to serve

Nutrition per serving:
Calories 529 | Total carbohydrate 11 g | Sugars 4 g | Fat 37 g
Protein 38 g | Sodium 672 mg

1. Start by trimming and then finely shredding the Brussels sprouts. Heat the olive oil in a non-stick sauté pan, then add the sprouts. Fry over a medium heat for 3–4 minutes until golden brown. Season and then add the butter and the chopped sage. Reduce the heat while you sort your eggs out.

2. In a bowl, whisk the eggs with the milk. Slice the ham and stir into the egg mix; season well.

3. Turn up the heat on your non-stick pan with the sprouts inside. Once sizzling, stir in the egg and ham mix. Continue to gently move the mix around over a high heat until the eggs start to firm up. Turn the heat down and continue cooking over a low heat for 2 minutes. Remove from the pan by folding over (flip with a spatula) and pour gently out of the pan onto a warmed plate. Serve with a big green salad.

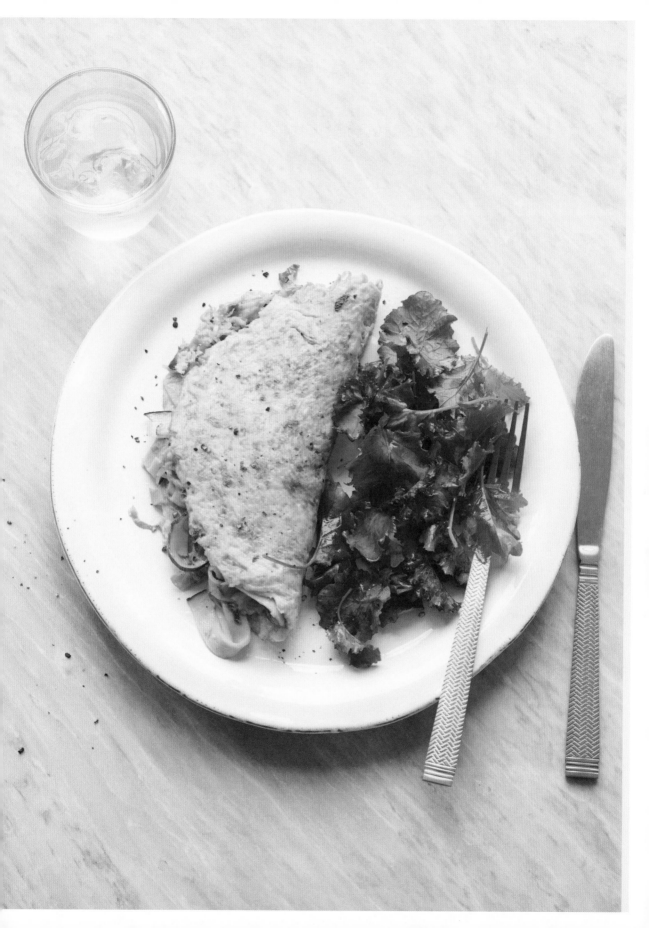

BBQ spiced sweet potato frittata

Try this for a solid meal, high in complex carbs and protein, ahead of a hard day on the bike. Any leftovers (unlikely!) are perfect for refuelling

This frittata contains really simple ingredients and can easily be made up in advance and reheated. If you are feeling flash, the addition of smoked bacon or spicy chorizo when cooking the sweet potatoes takes this to the next level. If you struggle to find a good BBQ spice, replace with a good-quality cajun spice – perhaps easier to find. There's no reason at all why you could not complete the whole dish in a non-stick baking tray.

Makes 2–3 portions

2 tablespoons olive oil

600 g (1 lb 5 oz) sweet potato, peeled and chopped

2 teaspoons BBQ spice mix

sea salt and freshly ground black pepper

8 large free-range eggs

Nutrition per serving:
Calories 479 | Total carbohydrate 43 g | Sugars 9 g | Fat 24 g
Protein 23 g | Sodium 425 mg

1 Preheat the oven to 200°C/400°F/Gas 6.

2. Place a large non-stick pan (ideally one with an ovenproof handle) over a medium heat. Warm the olive oil and add the sweet potato and BBQ spice and season well. Cook for 3–4 minutes until the sweet potato is golden brown.

3. Place the pan in the centre of the oven for 10 minutes until the potato is cooked. At this point, taste some potato: it should be soft and tender.

4 Whisk the eggs in a bowl, season and pour over the sweet potato mix. Place in the oven for 10–12 minutes. Allow to cool and firm up for 5 minutes, then slice into wedges and enjoy! This frittata is perfect served with a big green salad.

Huevos rancheros

This is quite calorific, but don't worry, there's still lots of good protein and carbs in there

I love the simplicity of this one-pan dish – there's something hugely satisfying about having posh fried eggs! It's perfect comfort food when you are feeling a little bit ruined after a hard ride.

Serves 2

120 g (4 oz) smoked chorizo

1 large red onion, peeled and sliced

1 green chilli, deseeded and finely sliced

200 g (7 oz) cooked baby new potatoes

4 medium free-range eggs

sea salt and freshly ground black pepper

2 spring onions, trimmed and sliced

a pinch of smoked paprika

Nutrition per serving:

Calories 549 | Total carbohydrate 28 g | Sugars 5 g
Fat 35 g | Protein 31 g | Sodium 2181 mg

1. Slice the chorizo into small chunks and place in a large non-stick sauté pan with the onion slices and chilli. Fry over a medium to low heat for 6–8 minutes. The fat from the chorizo should render down, which means there is no need to add any additional oil to the pan.

2. Add the potatoes (if you prefer, you can dice these up beforehand). Continue cooking over a medium heat for 3–4 minutes until the potatoes are golden brown.

3. Crack the eggs into the sauté pan and cook over a low heat for a further 4 minutes or until they are cooked. (You can also do this under the grill on a medium setting but make sure the chorizo/potato mix is evenly distributed throughout the base of the pan to allow for even cooking of the eggs.)

4. Season and finish off by sprinkling with spring onion slices and smoked paprika.

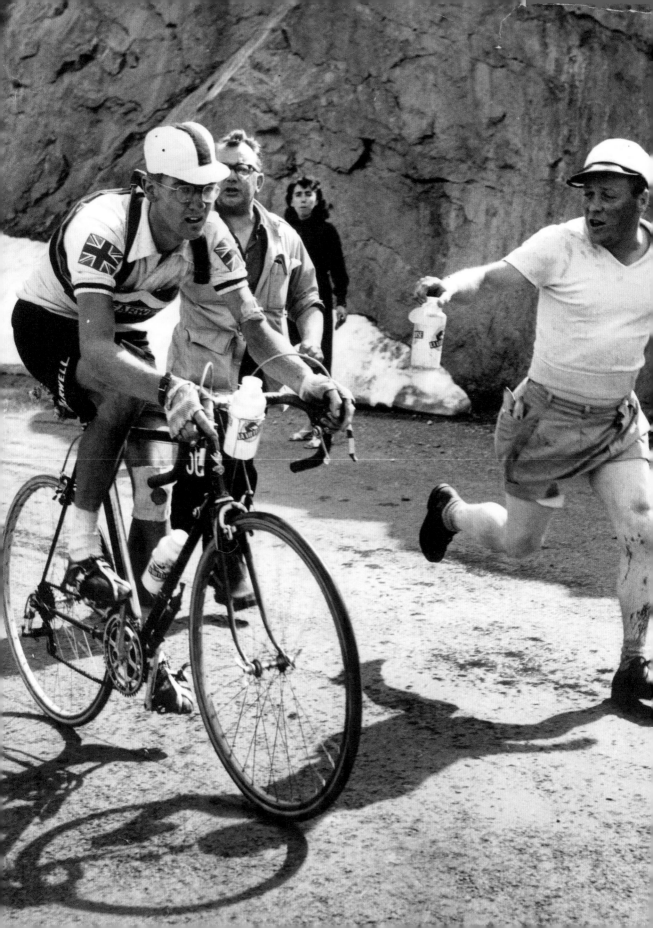

Nutrition and the Busy Life

Stop heading for the toaster or takeaway menu. Food and nutrition are often sacrificed by time-pressured cyclists eager to get on the bike, but being appropriately fuelled is just as vital as your training.

You've got a hectic life. Join the club! The way I see it is that if you are committed enough to put yourself through torment on two wheels, just for fun, then you've got the willpower to feed yourself properly too. The problems you face will most likely be the distractions of work, family and a social life, a lack of organisation and your psychological reactions to life's troubles – from hunger to heartbreak. All of these can be combatted through plenty of preparation and a little self-discipline.

Great Britain's Bob Maitland takes on supplies during the 1955 Tour de France. With all life's pressures and distractions, keeping to a nutrtional plan can sometimes prove difficult. Preparation and a little willpower will help you stay on track.

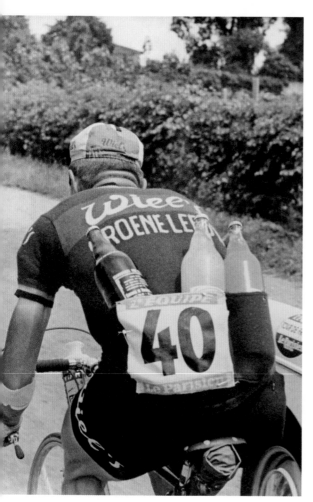

Belgian cyclist René Van Meenen carrying refreshments during the 1963 Tour de France. Getting nutrition on the go can be difficult so taking your own food on the road is the best way of controlling your diet.

Short-term planning is the key. Most of us have a fair idea of our commitments for the following week or so and will be able to gauge what we will need to buy. Shopping might be a chore but having the right food at home is the best way of avoiding the pitfalls of processed or junk food. Most of the store cupboard items (*see* p. 30) can be ordered online for delivery or topped up on a weekly supermarket trip, but you will need to buy fresh foods more regularly.

Mark out time to prepare meals too. Breakfast ingredients can be sorted in advance, and fruit and nut snacks distributed into small bags. Remember the importance of post-ride nutrition: cooking and eating might be the last things you want to do then so have something appetising ready prepared. Meals can be bulk-cooked and portioned in containers to keep in the fridge or freezer, but beware of repetition. Swap pulses, beans and grains; switch meat, chicken and fish in recipes, experiment with herbs and spices – variety is the best way of combatting boredom in your diet.

Enjoy being a 21st-century athlete and make the most of available technology. Slow cookers, oven timers and microwave ovens all mean meals can be ready when you need them, whether it's after a tough ride or an exhausting day at work. Rice cookers are super-convenient (and also work for quinoa and other grains) and smoothie blenders not only give you a nutritious meal in minutes, but are a speedy way of making soups and sauces. Finally, modern cool bags and flasks are pretty effective at keeping meals fresh or soups warm – ideal if you are taking lunch to work or need something to eat when travelling.

Although taking your own food with you on the road is the best way of controlling your diet, there will be times when this just isn't feasible so think carefully about your meal options. The budget high-street sandwich and pizza outlets are truly horrific nutritionally. Instead, consider small independent restaurants who offer good homemade food, or try sushi restaurants and noodle bars. Alternatively, go for the meal deal in your local supermarket, where sushi, a small bottle of fruit juice or a smoothie, and a raw fruit and nut bar are often available to buy together at a reasonable price.

We've all got our weaknesses. Be aware of them and be prepared to confront them. I try and travel with rice cakes, homemade energy bars, dried fruit and nuts in the car, knowing I will be less likely to graze on junk food. Use your phone or watch alarm as reminders to shop or cook, or even eat! And always have something prepared for when you really don't have the energy to cook. If you err, don't punish yourself. A night out eating curry, a chocolate binge or a takeaway is a blip. It happens. Accept it and start again. Don't over-train or skip meals to compensate, just concentrate on getting back to your plan.

Remember the importance of post-ride nutrition: cooking and eating might be the last things you want to do, so have something appetising ready prepared.

Lifestyle Rules

- Your dietary plan is as important as your training plan – stick to it.
- Plan meals and snacks and shop strategically.
- Allocate time to prepare meals as much in advance as possible.
- Give yourself time to eat – enjoy it; don't rush or leave food because you are in a hurry.
- Make use of slow cookers, microwaves, rice cookers and smoothie makers for easy prep, and cool bags and flasks for on-the-go food storage.
- Know your weaknesses and confront them. Crisps, chocolate and alcohol won't go away – deal with them. If you really struggle with this, consider seeking professional help from a doctor or registered sports nutritionist or dietician.
- Include travelling in your plans. Prepare snacks and meals for long journeys, or consider where you will eat.

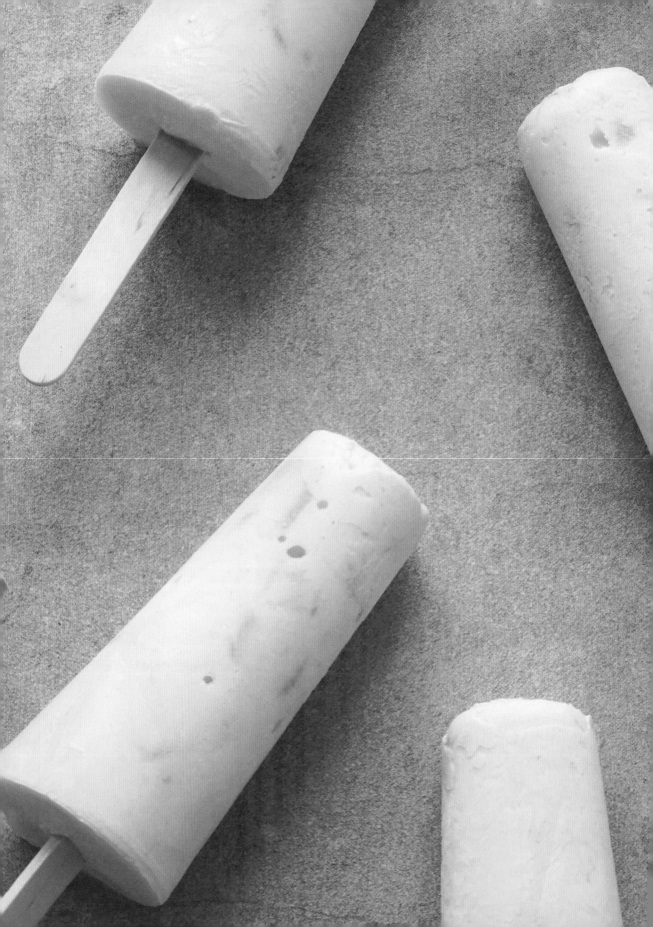

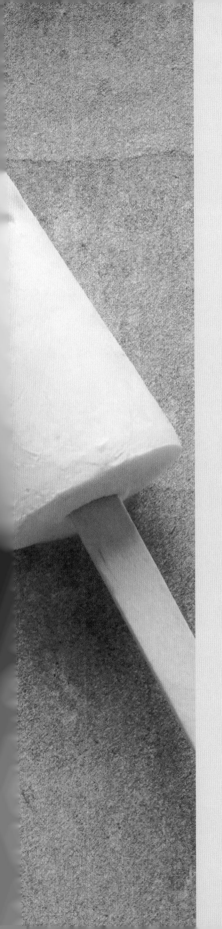

Smoothies and Snacks

The traditional three-meals-a-day structure doesn't match the fuel and recovery demands of the endurance athlete. Thankfully we have smoothies, energy bars and banana breads to see us through.

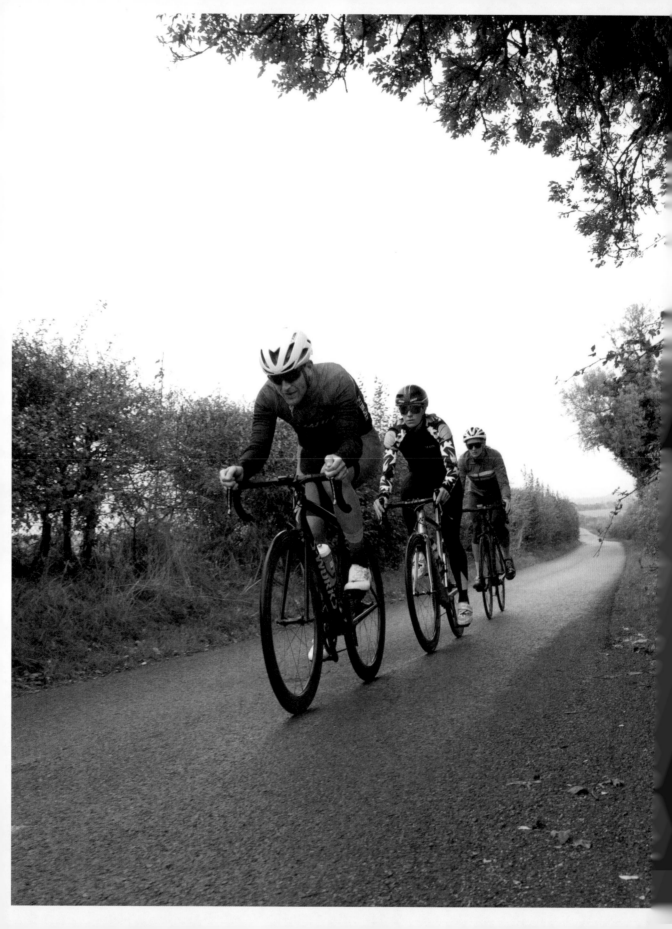

The smoothie has become the go-to convenience for 21st-century athletes. Throw some fruit and vegetables into a blender or smoothie machine and blitz until smooth. Simple and satisfying.

While you can't live on smoothies alone, a smoothie can serve as a lighter breakfast on an easy day with, say, blueberries, yogurt and honey; a blend of milk, banana and berries can provide a pre-race energy blast; and peanut butter and cocoa can be the basis of a post-ride recovery drink.

Others use the smoothie as a way of keeping on top of their fruit and veg intake. Vegetables such as kale, broccoli, chard, spinach and celery go down a treat when blitzed with mango, pineapple, orange, avocado and most other fruits. Stick to a ratio of around two cups of veg to three cups of fruit to two cups of liquid (try using dairy substitutes such as almond or coconut milk) and it should emerge in a drinkable state. I like to throw in a few ice cubes as this keeps the mix nice and cold – it can warm up due to the friction of the blades and no one wants a warm smoothie.

If it isn't already exciting enough, you can always super-charge your smoothie. Chia, hemp or flax seeds along with almonds or walnuts can boost your Omega-3 intake and provide a useful source of vitamins and minerals. If you have finished a long, tough ride or are in the middle of a stage race you might also consider adding a whey or similar protein powder to your recovery smoothie.

Convenient, nutritious, portable – what's not to like? Well, smoothies do sometimes get a bad press thanks to their high sugar content (from fruit sugars), but in all honesty, as part of a balanced diet, they are hard to criticise. If sugar is a concern then choose lower-sugar options such as frozen berries, kiwi fruit or avocado and ease up on the bananas, mangoes and pineapple.

Vegetables such as kale, broccoli, chard, spinach and celery go down a treat when blitzed with mango, pineapple, orange, avocado and most other fruits.

Club Tropicana… oh, and avocado?

This works really well as a meal replacement: the richness of the coconut milk and avocado truly adds another dimension

Perfect for when you are time poor, or want an easy-to-digest, highly nutritious 'meal' – maybe a couple of hours before a hard ride. If you are looking for a big old calorie hit, you can use regular canned coconut milk.

Serves 2

2 medium ripe avocados

400 ml (1 ½ cups) light coconut milk or coconut soya milk

250 ml (1 cup) pineapple juice

100 g (3 ½ oz) fresh or frozen mango

2 apples, skin on, cored and chopped

1 large banana, peeled

¼ fresh pineapple

juice of one lime

a handful of ice cubes

Nutrition per serving:
Calories 665 | Total carbohydrate 88.5 g
Sugars 60 g | Fat 34 g
Protein 7 g | Sodium 1400 mg

1. Simply place all the ingredients apart from the ice in a smoothie machine or blender and blitz until smooth. Serve with ice and enjoy ASAP!

Yellow mellow

This sunshine smoothie offers up anti-inflammatory properties, with a good kick of ginger to wake you up

A lovely morning smoothie to kickstart the day in a truly self-righteous way! High in vitamin C, with ginger to aid digestion, this is pretty much the perfect smoothie to keep your immune system in tip-top shape. If you can find fresh turmeric, please use it.

Serves 2

250 ml (1 cup) carrot juice

250 ml (1 cup) pineapple juice

100 g (3 ½ oz) pineapple

1 ripe banana, peeled

about 15 g (½ oz) fresh ginger, peeled

20 g cashews or 1 tablespoon cashew butter

1 tablespoon Manuka honey

a good pinch of turmeric

juice of half a lime

a handful of ice cubes

1. Place all the ingredients apart from the ice in a smoothie machine or blender and blitz until smooth. Serve with ice and enjoy ASAP!

Nutrition per serving:
Calories 270 | Total carbohydrate 55 g
Sugars 38 g | Fat 5 g
Protein 4 g | Sodium 1300 mg

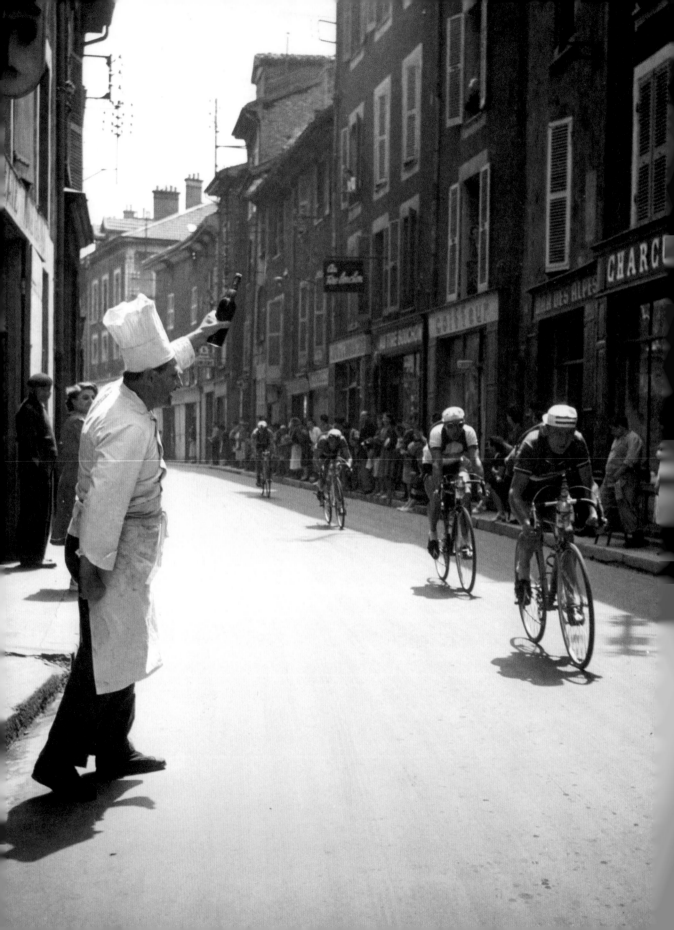

When to Eat, What to Eat

What an athlete consumes not only affects their short-term performance but also long-term health and fitness. Eating the right food at the right time is crucial.

OK, you're a sporting creature and you know how to eat healthily – plenty of fresh fruit and vegetables, keep the carbs under control, and avoid sugar and saturated fats as much as possible. Your doctor will be happy. But you are also an endurance athlete, which brings its own, sometimes conflicting, demands. Yes, you need to eat well, but you also need to eat specific food groups at specific times. Oh, and it's worth remembering you are an ordinary person too. You have a world outside cycling – family, work, friends – and face the stresses and temptations of everyday life. Somehow, you have to bring these worlds together.

A chef cheers on participants in the 1951 Tour de France as they speed past his restaurant. To be a successful endurance athlete, you need to eat well, but you also need to eat specific food groups at specific times.

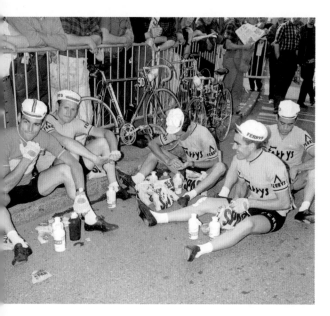

Antonio Bertran, Salvador Honrubia and Fernando Manzaneque of the Spanish road cycling team Ferrys rest and take on food at the 1964 Tour de France. During or immediately after your cool-down is the time to re-hydrate and take in carbohydrates, protein and electrolytes.

It's not that difficult, honestly. Eating good fresh food will still be the basis of your diet, just with some adjustments to allow for the demands you will place on your body. Cyclists are not normal (in many ways!) and if you compare a cyclist who is riding anything from 8–20 hours a week with a sedentary person then it would make sense to recognise that you are using more energy and require a lot more food to maintain health and well-being, let alone get any type of training benefit. We therefore have to look at how to keep you generally fit and healthy, how to fuel your rides and, just as importantly, how to replenish your body after you have pushed it to the limits.

You will find that on days when you are not riding, or you have a low-intensity ride, you can follow a pretty traditional structure of three meals a day. These days are still important, as by eating sensibly you can consume the necessary carbohydrates, proteins and fats to generate energy and muscle repair, and the vitamins and minerals that will provide long-term health and boost the immune system.

Breakfast (*see also* p. 40) is an opportunity to get some slow-release carbohydrates through oats or a piece of toast or eggs, which are a high source of protein. Lunch could be pasta, rice or a small bagel with some fish or chicken (turkey is also a great option) and some natural fat such as avocado. A light dinner could be vegetables with meat, fish, pulses or legumes. If you need to snack, go for a small handful of nuts and dried fruit (keep it small as these are high in calories) and keep clear of sugary, processed biscuits and sweets.

On harder training or race days things become a little more complicated. You will need to factor in a slow-releasing source of complex carbohydrates – such as wholegrain pasta or brown rice – two to three hours before any long session. If you are at work, think ahead and have a sandwich or some pre-cooked food ready. There's no real point in eating tons of pasta – just make sure you have a decent meal. However, around 30 minutes before a ride have a faster-releasing carbohydrate such as a banana to boost energy levels.

During a long ride you will need to replenish energy by eating on the bike. This is dealt with on pp. 154–159, so let's skip to the end of the ride. The muscles' ability to process and store nutrients increases after exercise, so during or immediately after your cool-down is the time to re-hydrate and take in carbohydrates, protein and electrolytes. This might most easily be achieved through a smoothie (*see also* p. 142. However, do not wait long before refuelling with solid food. Chicken, eggs or lentils can provide valuable protein to repair muscle damage, and wholegrains, rice and vegetables can help restock glycogen stores.

Finally, a word of warning about eating out before an event. A wise man once said 'a chef should never be left with your girlfriend, your car or your kitchen as there's a very good chance they will never be the same again'. The reason food tastes so good in restaurants is that chefs incorporate copious amounts of salt, butter, cream, cheese and more into their dishes. The quality of the protein and carbohydrate that they are serving up can vary hugely and the calorie and fat content in the dishes you eat in a restaurant can be massive. Don't let a chef with an ego (they *all* have egos!) be the undoing of your key event. So often when cyclists under-perform in races it comes down to the food they have eaten the night before the race.

If you do need to eat out pre-event then choose tactically with safe foods that you know and recognise – leave the experimental cuisine until you have passed the finish line!

Eating Rules

- Eat real food. The body processes nutrients from wholefoods, whether that is meat, fish, fruit, veg or grains, most effectively.
- Eat optimally. Match the training load with appropriate fuelling.
- Eat protein – around 1.5–2 grams per kilo of body weight every day, to aid muscle recovery. Nuts, milk, olive oil, avocados, fish and even a little fat on your red meat all provide a natural mix of saturated and unsaturated fats.
- Cyclists need sugar and natural sugars found in fruit should be a part of any healthy balanced diet. Try where possible to use honey or maple syrup in place of refined white sugar. Never ever eat or drink anything that has fake sugar – better to have a full sugar product and get over it.
- Be snack smart. Training sessions don't always fit neatly between meal times. Snack on energy bars, muffins, nuts and berries. (*See also* p. 154.)
- Cheese is awesome but also the work of the Devil! Parmesan or Grana Padano are very good grated on top of dishes to give you a cheese hit with a lower calorie content.
- A glass of beer or wine might help you relax, but it's calories without nutrients. It's not going to get you fitter or faster!
- Simple water is the most important nutrient in your body. Don't take it for granted – hydrate yourself throughout the day and after a ride.

Nutty slack

For me, this is the ultimate protein recovery smoothie: a staple in our household

Milk, oats, nuts, banana, honey… and boom! Simple, effective, tasty and very easy to digest, post-ride you can't go far wrong with this. Whey protein is a supplement that can help boost your overall protein intake and provides essential amino acids to promote muscle growth and repair. Always look out for the 'informed sports' logo on the product you choose. This is absolutely essential for any serious competing cyclist. It guarantees that the protein powder has not been contaminated with other supplements that could result in a positive doping test.

Serves 2

500 ml (2 cups) milk (either cow's milk or unsweetened almond milk)

20 g (¾ oz) gluten-free oats

20 g (¾ oz) Brazil nuts

1 teaspoon ground cinnamon

2 tablespoons almond or peanut butter

20 g (¾ oz) honey

1 ripe banana, peeled

50 g (2 oz) whey protein powder

a handful of ice cubes

Nutrition per serving:
Calories 518 | Total carbohydrate 43 g
Sugars 28 g | Fat 23 g
Protein 35 g | Sodium 40 mg

1. Place all the ingredients apart from the ice in a smoothie machine or blender and blitz until smooth. Serve with ice and enjoy ASAP!

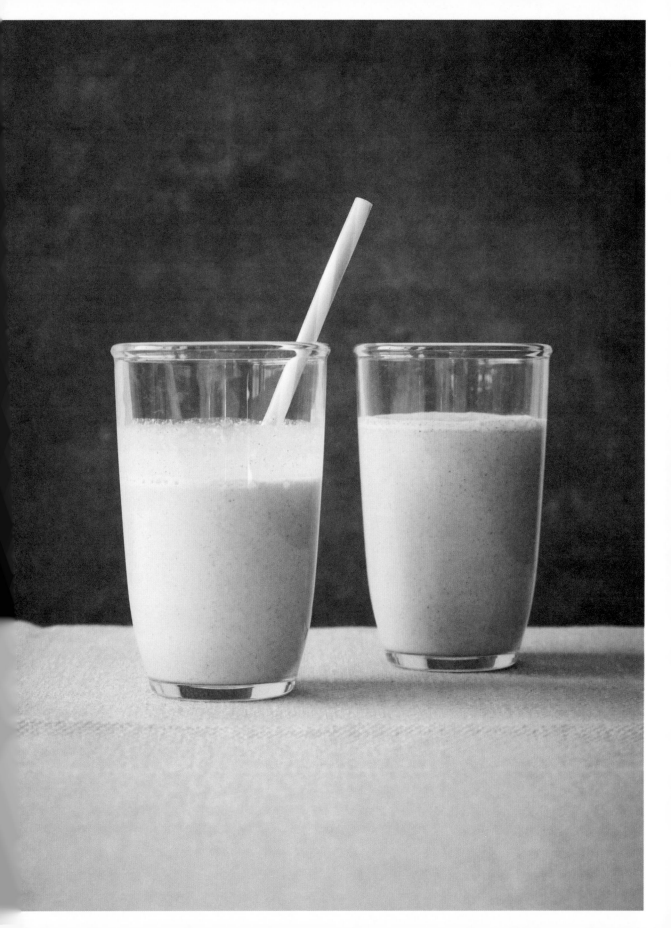

Nitrate turbo booster

Beetroot juice is a well-documented source of nitrates, which increase the transportation of oxygen to the blood

Despite its worthiness, beetroot juice can taste pretty rank on its own! But by incorporating frozen blueberries and a hit of concentrated cherry juice, we can make it taste great. A dash of apple juice and some Greek yoghurt rounds things off nicely.

Serves 2

300 ml (1 ¼ cups) beetroot juice

300 ml (1 ¼ cups) apple juice

2 apples, cored and chopped

200 g (7 oz) frozen blueberries (or you can use frozen mixed berries)

2 ripe bananas, peeled

2 tablespoons Greek yoghurt

1 tablespoon chia seeds

1 tablespoon concentrated cherry juice

a handful of ice cubes

1. Place all the ingredients apart from the ice in a smoothie machine or blender and blitz until smooth. Serve with ice and enjoy ASAP!

Nutrition per serving:
Calories 453 | Total carbohydrate 100 g
Sugars 65 g | Fat 4 g
Protein 7 g | Sodium 800 mg

Supergreens smoothie

A real kickstart to the day! This one is great if, for whatever reason, you haven't been able to eat lots of fruit and veggies

We always try to incorporate greens into every main meal in my house. However, I'm aware that sometimes this is not possible for a time-crunched cyclist balancing work, family and training commitments, so this smoothie is a great way to get some green veg in with no bother. You can add an avocado to this smoothie if you want to make it richer and more calorie-dense. If you are making this recipe in advance, add some crushed ice just before serving – it needs to be nice and cold.

Serves 2–3

400 ml (1 ½ cups) apple juice

4 kiwi fruit, skin on

40 green seedless grapes

2 ripe bananas, peeled

2 green apples, skin on, cored

a handful of fresh spinach

a handful of fresh kale

1 tablespoon flax seeds

a handful of ice cubes

Nutrition per serving:
Calories 324 | Total carbohydrate 73 g
Sugars 42 g | Fat 2 g
Protein 3 g | Sodium 105 mg

1. Place all the ingredients apart from the ice into a smoothie machine or blender and blitz until smooth. Serve with ice and enjoy ASAP!

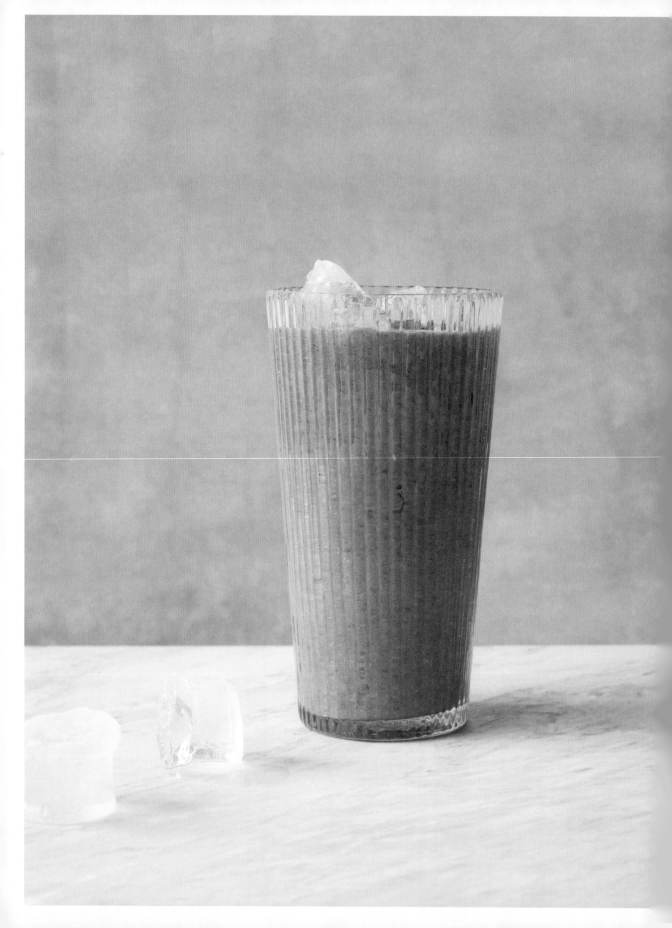

Maca-matcha smoothie

A bit of a healthy one this, with lots of good stuff going on!

Maca is high in antioxidants, minerals and B vitamins and is also a good source of iron for vegans. A teaspoon of maca powder provides 10 per cent of your daily iron needs. Matcha helps boost metabolism, enhances mood and encourages concentration. It has 10 times the antioxidant levels of green tea (which we all know tastes like grass!)

Makes 1 large self-righteous smoothie

250 ml (1 cup) almond milk

2 teaspoons maca powder

1 teaspoon matcha powder

1 teaspoon flaxseed

a pinch of cinnamon

2 Medjool dates

1 ripe banana, peeled

a handful of spinach

1 tablespoon almond butter

a handful of ice

Nutrition per serving:
Calories 478 | Total carbohydrate 88 g
Sugars 59 g | Fat 13 g
Protein 13 g | Sodium 25 mg

1. Simply place all the ingredients apart from the ice in a smoothie machine or blender and blitz until smooth. Serve with ice and enjoy ASAP!

Snack like a pro

Snacking carries some pretty negative connotations. All those eating-between-meals warnings and guilt trips associated with devouring chocolate bars and packets of crisps. It's true that snacking is the downfall of many a cyclist: you can eat really well at main meal times but then undo all that good work by eating sub-optimal food in between. However, there is also a place for planned snacking. You might well include a smoothie, a handful of seeds and dried fruit, some roasted chickpeas or even a mid-afternoon bagel in your nutritional plan.

That unforeseen snack attack is still going to happen, though. The best we can do is prepare for it by making our own healthy snacks. Most of these recipes would work well in response to that mid-morning energy dip, as a boost two to three hours ahead of an evening bike session, or as a healthy dessert when served with some Greek yoghurt.

It is also crucial that you 'fuel the machine' when you're actually on the bike. For rides of anything up to an hour, you don't need to take a picnic with you. But when it comes to longer rides or any type of ride that burns lots of glycogen (muscle fuel), you will need to eat along the way. There are so many commercially available products out there, and there is a time and a place for such things, but why not try making your own snacks up? It's a fairly simple rest-day job that you can do once a week. This is real food and you know exactly what goes into it – and it's more cost-effective than those pre-packaged bars!

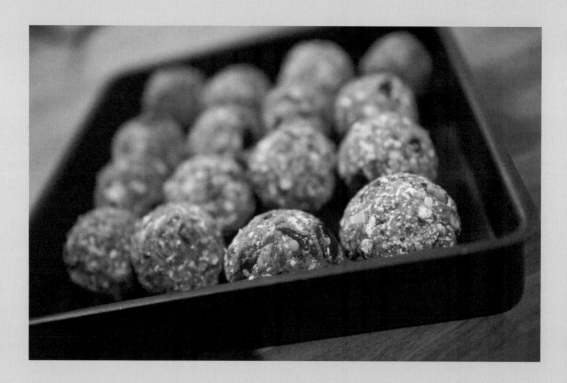

Bitter chocolate and sweet potato brownies

Sweet potatoes are a rich source of vitamin A, and pack in twice as much dietary fibre as their white cousins

Two of my favourite foods in one place! As we all know, high-cocoa-content chocolate is actually very good for you too. Also, an interesting fact: botanically, the sweet potato belongs to the 'Morning Glory' family. It just gets better all the time…

Makes 20 good-sized brownies

1 tablespoon coconut oil

450 g (1 lb) sweet potatoes, peeled and diced

2 teaspoons ground cinnamon

Himalayan salt and freshly ground black pepper

50 g (2 oz) Manuka honey

180 g (6 oz) unsalted butter, diced

200 g (7 oz) chocolate (70 per cent cocoa solids), melted

50 g (2 oz) brown sugar

4 large eggs

200 g (7 oz) plain flour

1 teaspoon baking powder

1 tablespoon cocoa powder

100 g (3 ½ oz) walnuts

1 tablespoon chia seeds

vegetable or olive oil spray

Nutrition per serving:

Calories 257 | Total carbohydrate 22 g | Sugars 8 g
Fat 17 g | Protein 5 g | Sodium 52 mg

1. Gently heat the coconut oil in a non-stick sauté pan. Add the diced sweet potatoes, cinnamon and seasoning. Cook over a medium heat until the potatoes have some nice colour and have softened (allow about 6–8 minutes). Stir in the honey and set aside to cool for 10 minutes.

2. Place the sweet potato mix in the bowl of a food processor and slowly add the butter, melted chocolate and brown sugar. Blend for 60 seconds, then add the eggs.

3. The next stage is to blend in the flour, baking powder and cocoa powder; ensure the flour is mixed in well. Last, but not least, stir in the walnuts and chia seeds. Ensure you don't overblend the walnuts as you want to keep the texture of the nuts.

4. Preheat the oven to 180°C/350°F/Gas 4. Pour the mixture evenly into a lined non-stick baking tray (line with greaseproof paper and spray with a little oil) and bake for 20 minutes. Allow to cool for at least 15 minutes (if you can resist) and then slice into chunks. Once cooled, store in an airtight box in the fridge for up to a week.

Warm avocado, chocolate and pistachio cookies

Healthy cookies are now officially a real thing! Perfect for when you want to recharge on a ride

These are best served warm and also make a great dessert topped with some natural yoghurt. The recipe makes quite a lot of cookies so I suggest you freeze 50 per cent of the mix to avoid the temptation of eating them all at once. Shape half the raw mixture into a sausage shape approximately 10 cm long and wrap in cling film. This will keep for up to a month in the freezer. For an easy snack, cook straight from frozen by removing the cling film and slicing into rounds 2 cm in thickness. When cooking straight from frozen, add 2 minutes on to the cooking time.

Makes 24 cookies

25 g (1 oz) cocoa nibs (Grue de Cacao)

200 g (7 oz) ripe avocado flesh

75 g (3 oz) organic cocoa powder

2 medium eggs

100 g (3 ½ oz) gluten-free plain flour

2 teaspoons baking powder

180 g (6 oz) Manuka honey

150 g (5 oz) chocolate (70 per cent cocoa solids), chopped into chunks

75 g (3 oz) whole pistachio nuts

Nutrition per serving:

Calories 199 | Total carbohydrate 22 g | Sugars 12 g
Fat 11 g | Protein 5 g | Sodium 38 mg

1. Preheat the oven to 180°C/350°F/Gas 4. Meanwhile, place the cocoa nibs in the bowl of a food processor and blend until a fine powder forms. Add the avocado flesh and cocoa powder and blend again into a smooth paste.

2. Add the eggs, flour, baking powder and honey. Incorporate well until you have a smooth dough.

3. Stir the chocolate chunks into the avocado mix, along with the pistachios.

4. The mixture will be quite wet so you will find it tricky to mould. Instead, use a spoon to place dollops of cookie dough on a non-stick baking sheet (about 90 mm / 3.5 inch in width and 30 mm / 1 inch deep). Bake in the centre of the oven for 7–8 minutes. Allow to cool for 5 minutes on the tray before getting stuck in!

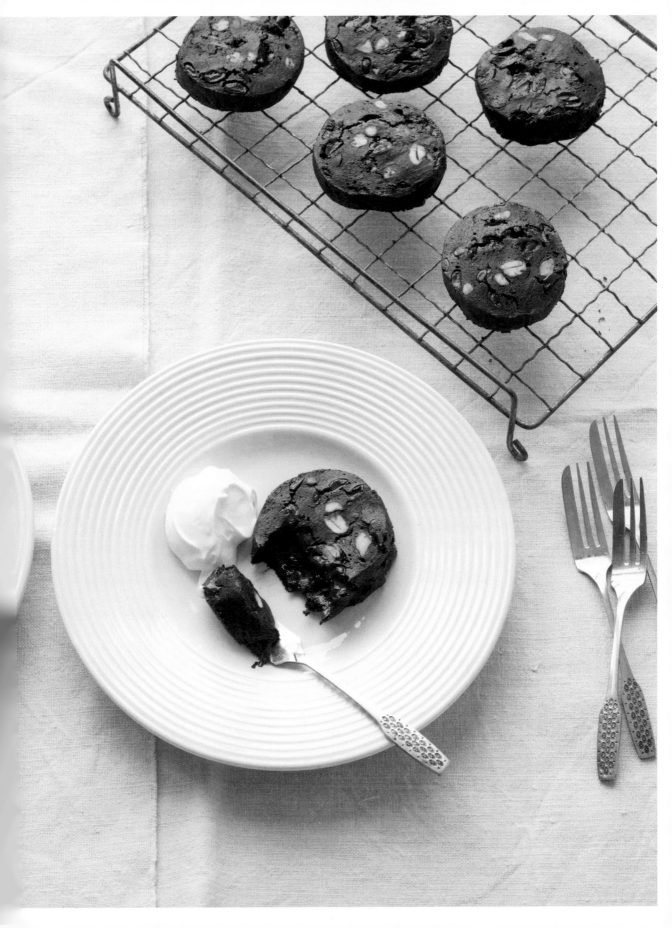

Parsnip, coconut and banana bread

Perfect for long rides, bananas contain potassium to help replace the electrolytes lost through sweating

A slightly savoury element is good for a change and here, the flavour profiles of parsnip and coconut work so well together. It's also great for using up overripe bananas. Once your bananas are past their best, store them in the freezer, still in their skins, to intensify the flavour. If you don't own a food mixer, you can easily follow the same process in a food processor – it is literally a bombproof recipe!

Makes 1 medium loaf

250 g (9 oz) ripe bananas

200 g (7 oz) brown sugar

150 g (5 oz) grated parsnip

2 eggs

25 g (1 oz) blackstrap molasses

35 g (1 ½ oz) desiccated coconut (1 tablespoon for sprinkling, if liked)

250 g (9 oz) strong flour

a pinch of sea salt

14 g (½ oz) baking powder

25 ml (1 ½ tablespoons) olive oil

50 ml (3 tablespoons) milk

100 g (3 ½ oz) chocolate (70 per cent cocoa solids)

Nutrition per serving:
Calories 205 | Total carbohydrate 32 g | Sugars 18 g | Fat 7 g
Protein 4 g | Sodium 166 mg

1 Preheat the oven to 180°C/350°F/Gas 4.

2. In the bowl of a food mixer, and using the paddle attachment, beat the bananas, brown sugar and grated parsnip together for 5 minutes. Add the eggs and the molasses and beat for a further 2 minutes.

3. Next, add the coconut, flour, sea salt and baking powder. Beat for a further minute until the dry goods are well incorporated.

4. Whisk the oil and the milk together in a separate bowl and add to the mix.

5. Line a 22 cm x 22 cm (9 inch x 9 inch) baking tin with greaseproof paper and spray with a little olive oil. Fold the chocolate into the cake mix and pour into the tin. At this point it is nice to sprinkle a tablespoon of desiccated coconut over the cake mix, as you will get a nice toasted coconut flavour as it cooks. Place in the centre of the oven and bake for 35–40 minutes. Leave to cool in the tin for 5–10 minutes and then transfer to a wire rack to finish cooling.

Mocha and date 'buzzing' bars

A good hit of caffeine and the richness of chocolate to boost your energy levels

You can increase the amount of coffee in this recipe if you prefer a stronger coffee taste. Use the best-quality instant coffee granules you can find. It's probably best to avoid these bars before bed due to the caffeine!

Makes 10 x 50 g (2 oz) bars

150 g (5 oz) cocoa nibs (Grue de Cacao)

75 g (3 oz) almonds

75 g (3 oz) walnuts

150 g (5 oz) Medjool dates

50 g (2 oz) raisins

6 g (¼ oz) dried espresso powder (up to 10 g / ½ oz depending on taste, any more than this and it will become too bitter)

2 tablespoons sesame seeds

Nutrition per serving:

Calories 260 | Total carbohydrate 21 g | Sugars 14 g
Fat 18 g | Protein 5.5 g | Sodium 1.4 mg

1. Blend the cocoa nibs to a fine powder in a food processor. Add the nuts and repeat the process: do not overwork the nuts as the oil will split out of them, which will make the bars greasy.

2. Now add the dates, raisins and espresso powder; blend until the mix comes together.

3. Line a 22 cm x 22 cm (9 inch x 9 inch) baking tray with greaseproof paper and spray with a little olive oil. Press the mixture into the tray and sprinkle with sesame seeds. With your fingertips, press the seeds firmly on to the mix. Place in the fridge for 60 minutes, then cut into 50 g (2 oz) bars. These bars will keep well in the fridge for up to 2 weeks.

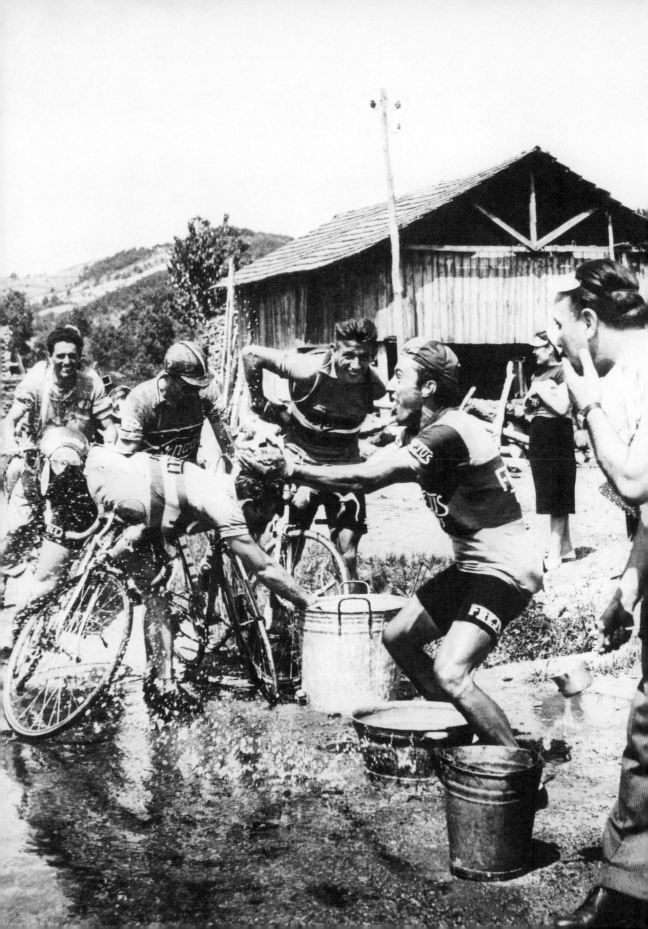

Training Camps

A training camp can be a perfect way to kick-start your cycling season, but a week or two of intensive riding has its own fuelling implications.

Training camps are an increasingly popular option for high-performance cyclists looking to intensify their training. At a camp, away from work or family commitments, it is perfectly possible to double your training load. Often this involves riding on challenging terrain in warmer or more humid climates. In an unfamiliar situation, it is all too easy for riders who stick to their usual food and fluid intakes to find themselves dehydrated or in energy deficit. It is therefore important to assess your fuelling and hydration strategy. Make sure you are familiar with the training schedule. Organised camps usually increase the intensity after a couple of days, have a rest day before another tough ride and then taper the week out.

Tour de France competitors drench themselves in an attempt to cool down in the intense summer heat. Training camps are unfamiliar situations and it is all too easy for riders who stick to their usual food and fluid intakes to find themselves dehydrated or in energy deficit.

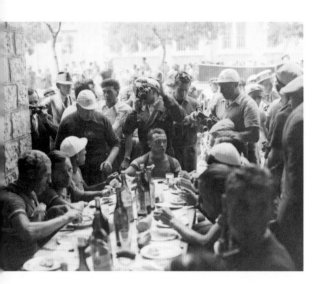

The 1950s Unis Sport team enjoying lunch during the Tour de France. When attending training camps try to resist the all-you-can-eat-style buffet or tempting desserts and pastries. Remember, you have come on a training camp, not a biking holiday.

The extra riding you are doing could well test your levels of fitness. Remember to stay hydrated – on and off the bike. If the weather is hot you could be losing fluid even walking around the camp during rest periods. Drink little and often, alternating between water and electrolyte drinks. Eating properly is even more essential when your training increases in intensity. If you are tired, it is all too easy to try to keep going with caffeine, gel or sugar boosts. This might get you through a ride but it could also ruin your training, so eat real food and take a rest day if necessary.

Depending on the location of your training camp you might wish to be cautious over drinking tap water. It may be fine for locals who are used to drinking it, but visitors might not have the same tolerance. A supply of bottled water could be a worthwhile investment if it keeps your digestive system healthy. Beware too any salad or other raw foods that have been washed in water that could cause an upset stomach.

What you are able to eat may depend upon what is provided by the organisers. Usually there will be a choice and you will be wise to stick to what you know. When you are tired and have another ride scheduled in the morning, it really isn't the time to be experimenting with local specialities or anything else that might be unfamiliar. The dining table is a good place to discuss dietary strategies, but don't be led astray by others in your group. If you are going to reconsider your plan, wait until you return home.

The other danger is that you over-fuel. Even if you can resist the urge to return to the all-you-can-eat-style buffet often provided at training camps, it can still be difficult to judge the portion sizes you are used to at home. There could well be tempting desserts on offer too and you might find pastries laid out in the morning spread. Stick to the oat-based breakfasts that will help see you through the morning ride. After all, you have come on a training camp, not a biking holiday – you'd be surprised how many cyclists return home weighing more than when they set out.

You should also take your own commercially made energy gels along with you. There might be none available locally or, although some organisers provide them, a different brand may disagree with you. This is not the time to try something new. If you are self-catering at your camp consider you might also need to take supplies with you to maintain health and energy levels. If you will have difficulty buying fresh produce then consider packing extra protein powder (fill a zip-lock bag if you don't want to take a whole container) in your suitcase and remember some spices and seasonings – just because you're cooking away from home there is no need to scrimp on flavour.

Finally, include any travelling time in your plans. When travelling by plane factor in at least eight hours door-to-door and take appropriate food and drink with you, paying particular attention to your hydration. Do all you can to ensure you hit the road fit and fully fuelled. Similarly, plan ahead for the return trip. Ensure you have enough sweet and savoury provisions such as muffins, fruit and bagels for the journey and that you are able to eat something nourishing when you arrive home.

Training Camp Tips

- Use camp to reinforce good nutrition habits.
- Take personal responsibility for your fuelling – don't rely on camp organisers.
- Adapt food and fluid intake according to training load.
- Pay careful attention to post-ride recovery in multi-day training situations.
- Beware the buffet – avoid over-eating and drinking, especially desserts, pastries and alcohol.
- Take your own energy gels and any multivitamins.
- Stick to familiar foods – avoid local delicacies.
- Ensure you have appropriate provisions for travel time, including transfers and potential delays.
- Remember to stay hydrated before, during and after any flight. Avoid caffeine and alcohol as both promote dehydration. Because of airport regulations you may need to buy water once you have cleared the security gates.

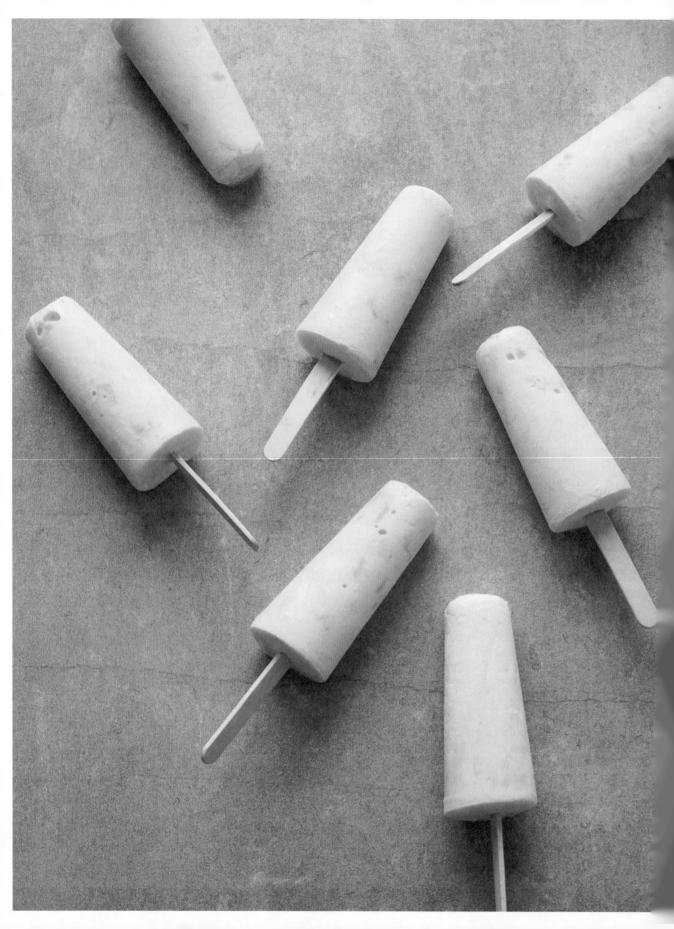

Mango and pineapple rehydrate lollies

A unique and refreshing way of replacing lost salts and aiding recovery after a hard ride on a hot day

A genius idea of mine, this one! Electrolyte tabs are a convenient way of replacing minerals lost through sweat. They have been formulated by leading sports scientists and are an easy and effective solution to fight dehydration during summer riding or indoor training sessions. You can get them online or from sports stores, health food shops and some supermarkets. High protein yoghurt adds more bang for your buck than standard yoghurt and scores your muscles recovery brownie points.

Makes 8–10

2 electrolyte tablets (preferably mango, pineapple or citrus flavour)

250 ml (1 cup) pineapple juice

500 g (1 lb 2 oz) high-protein yoghurt

1 mango, peeled, stone removed and finely diced

zest of 1 lime

1 tablespoon Manuka honey

a pinch of sea salt

1. Start by dissolving the electrolyte tablets in the pineapple juice. Then mix the yoghurt with the mango flesh, lime zest, honey and sea salt in a bowl before whisking in the pineapple juice mix.

2. Pour into ice lolly moulds and freeze for 2–3 hours. They will keep in the freezer for 3 months.

Nutrition per serving:
Calories 42 | Total carbohydrate 9 g | Sugars 8 g | Fat 0.1 g
Protein 1 g | Sodium 100 mg

Tropical rice pudding

A big dessert as a reward for a big day on the bike

This rice pudding eats well hot or cold, so could easily be prepared in advance and devoured after a bike ride.

Serves 3–4

100 g (3 ½ oz) basmati rice

1 tin (400 ml / 1 ½ cups) coconut milk

2 tablespoons honey

1 teaspoon vanilla extract

150 g (5 oz) fresh pineapple

100 g (3 ½ oz) fresh mango

2 passion fruit

1 teaspoon grated lime zest

1 tablespoon toasted coconut

Nutrition per serving:
Calories 240 | Total carbohydrate 38 g | Sugars 14 g | Fat 9 g
Protein 4 g | Sodium 9 mg

1. Combine the basmati rice with the coconut milk, honey and vanilla in a medium saucepan. Simmer over a low heat for about 10–14 minutes. The time can vary depending on the brand of rice, so keep an eye on the rice during cooking and add more water if necessary.

2. As the rice is cooking, prepare the fruit. Lay the pineapple on its side on a large chopping board. Hold it steady and with a sharp knife, remove the base. Now hold it upright by the leaves and slice away the skin from top to bottom. Remove the core and the leaves before slicing into chunks. If you have a blowtorch, you can be extra-fancy and char the pineapple chunks for extra flavour. Remove the skin and stone from the mango, then dice. Slice the passion fruit in half and scoop out the edible seeds and skin.

3. When the rice has absorbed the coconut milk and is tender, set aside for 5 minutes. Transfer to bowls and top with the tropical fruit, lime zest and toasted coconut.

Baked figs with quark

Think of this as a muscle repair dessert!

Quark is hugely popular in Scandinavia, with good reason: it is a really excellent source of protein, with double the protein levels of Greek yoghurt at 14 per cent. Here, the richness of quark works really well with the sweetness of the figs.

Serves 2

6 medium fresh figs

1 tablespoon honey

½ teaspoon cinnamon

a pinch of freshly ground black pepper

2 tablespoons quark

1 tablespoon pine nuts

1 teaspoon pumpkin seeds

1. Preheat the oven to 190°C/375°F/Gas 5. Slice the figs in half and place in an ovenproof dish.

2. Spoon the honey over the figs, sprinkle with cinnamon and freshly ground black pepper. Place the dish in the centre of the oven to bake for 10 minutes.

3. Allow to cool, then serve with the quark, pine nuts and pumpkin seeds. Spoon over the honey from the baking dish too.

Nutrition per serving:

Calories 228 | Total carbohydrate 43 g | Sugars 35 g | Fat 5 g
Protein 4 g | Sodium 3 mg

Mia's cherry go-go

A great way to satisfy your hunger pangs and full of dietary fibre, protein and good fats

Mia is my youngest daughter and a bit of a live wire, with a sweet tooth and a love of chocolate. We developed this recipe together and the collaboration satisfied both parties: she got to eat chocolate and I got her to make me some healthy bike snacks! Win-win…

Makes 14 x 40 g (1 ½ oz) balls

150 g (5 oz) cocoa nibs (Grue de Cacao)

80 g (3 oz) walnuts

35 g (1 ½ oz) almonds

35 g (1 ½ oz) Brazil nuts

150 g (5 oz) raisins

50 g (2 oz) glacé cherries

50 g (2 oz) dried sweetened cherries

Nutrition per serving:

Calories 195 | Total carbohydrate 17 g | Sugars 12 g
Fat 12.5 g | Protein 3 g | Sodium 1 mg

1. Place the cocoa nibs in the bowl of a food processor and blitz to a fine powder. Add the nuts and repeat the process, grinding to a fine powder. Don't overwork the nuts or the oil will split out of them, which will make the finished product greasy.

2. Add the raisins and both types of cherries and blend until a dry paste is formed. On a board, roll the paste with your hands into 40 g (1 ½ oz) balls, then store in the fridge for up to 2 weeks.

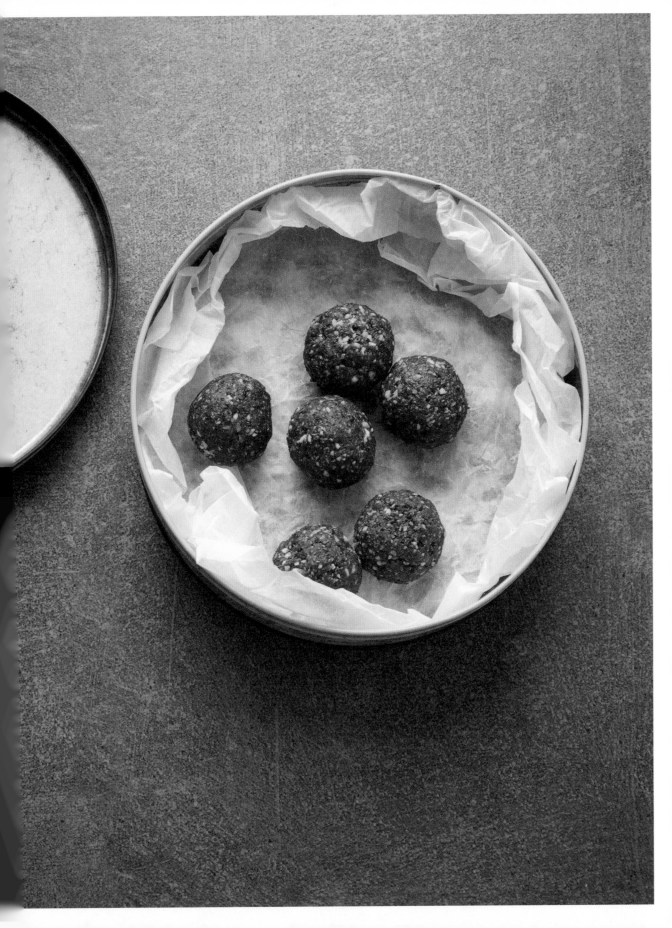

Budgie cage bars

All these ingredients are here for a good purpose, as seeds and nuts are high in protein and also loaded with good fats

So many seeds, it looks like the bottom of a budgie's cage! This recipe is my partner Vicky's speciality – if she can make these, anyone can! I have developed this really simple bar that can be used on the bike to prevent the hunger knock or as a pick-me-up between meals. It contains a mix of quick and slow release carbs and good fats, but most importantly of all, these bars taste banging!

Makes 16 x 50 g (2 oz) bars

280 g (10 oz) Medjool dates

65 g (2 ½ oz) Manuka honey

a pinch of Himalayan salt

80 g (3 oz) almond or peanut butter

90 g (3 ½ oz) Brazil nuts

50 g (2 oz) hazelnuts, skin on

20 g (¾ oz) flax seeds

60 g (2 ½ oz) chia seeds

3 teaspoons sunflower seeds

20 g (¾ oz) sesame seeds

3 teaspoons pumpkin seeds

40 g (1 ½ oz) puffed quinoa (this is like posh Rice Krispies!)

1 teaspoon vanilla extract

50 g (2 oz) vanilla protein powder

1. Place the dates and honey in the bowl of a mixer fitted with the paddle attachment. Beat slowly to form a coarse paste.

2. Add the remaining ingredients. Slowly mix together until a dry paste forms and all the ingredients are evenly incorporated. If the mix is too dry, add more honey and if it is too wet, add some more protein powder. You should be able to shape the mix into balls without it sticking to your hands.

3. Line a 22 cm x 22 cm (9 inch x 9 inch) baking tray with greaseproof paper and spray with a little olive oil. Press the mix into the tray and place in the fridge for 1½ hours to firm up before slicing into 50 g (2 oz) bars. Store in an airtight container in the fridge for up to 2 weeks.

Nutrition per serving:

Calories 218 | Total carbohydrate 21 g | Sugars 15 g
Fat 12 g | Protein 7 g | Sodium 105 mg

Spicy ginger and coconut bars

The Medjool dates in this one ensure you are getting a good source of energy, as they are loaded with glucose

Ginger and coconut is a classic combo and these bars also have a bit of a savoury element with the addition of the Himalyan salt, freshly ground black pepper and turmeric. A lovely dessert can be made by chopping up one bar (50 g / 2 oz) and adding to some Greek yoghurt with a teaspoon of honey.

Makes 16 x 50 g (2 oz) bars

250 g (9 oz) Medjool dates

200 g (7 oz) raisins

75 g (3 oz) whole almonds

250 g (9 oz) walnuts

75 g (3 oz) desiccated coconut

80 g (3 oz) crystallised stem ginger, finely chopped

1 teaspoon dried ginger powder

a pinch of Himalayan salt

a pinch of freshly ground black pepper

3 teaspoons ground cinnamon

a pinch of dried turmeric

Nutrition per serving:

Calories 269 | Total carbohydrate 24 g | Sugars 24 g
Fat 16 g | Protein 4 g | Sodium 28 mg

1. Place the dates and raisins in the bowl of a mixer fitted with the paddle attachment. Beat slowly to form a coarse paste.

2. Add the remaining ingredients and slowly mix together until a dry paste forms and all the ingredients are evenly incorporated. If the mix is too dry, add more honey and if it is too wet, add some more coconut. You should be able to form the mix into balls without it sticking to your hands.

3. Line a 22 cm x 22 cm (9 inch x 9 inch)baking tray with greaseproof paper and spray with a little olive oil. Press the mix into the tray and place in the fridge for 1½ hours to firm up before slicing into 50 g (2 oz) bars. Store in an airtight container in the fridge for up to 2 weeks.

Banana, chocolate and puffed quinoa energy bars

The naturally dried banana and sweet dried prunes here are both great for aiding digestion

Chocolate with 100 per cent cocoa solids gives a much more interesting savoury element to these energy bars.

Makes 28 x 50 g (2 oz) bars

250 g (9 oz) naturally dried banana

450 g (1 lb) Medjool dates

70 g (2 ½ oz) dried prunes

100 g (3 ½ oz) organic puffed quinoa

80 g (3 oz) organic banana powder

a pinch of Himalayan sea salt

125 g (4 oz) dried banana slices

100 g (3 ½ oz) chocolate (100 per cent cocoa solids), cut into chunks

130 g whole almonds

1 large vanilla pod (scrape the seeds from inside) or 1 teaspoon vanilla extract

60 g (2 ½ oz) maple syrup

1. Place the dried banana, dates and prunes in the bowl of a food mixer fitted with the paddle attachment. Beat slowly until all the ingredients are combined and you have a coarse paste.

2. Incorporate the remaining ingredients slowly, ensuring the dry goods are thoroughly mixed in.

3. Line a 22 cm x 22 cm (9 inch x 9 inch) baking tray with greaseproof paper and spray with a little olive oil. Press the mix into the tray and place in the fridge for 2–3 hours until set. Slice into 50 g (2 oz) bars and enjoy! These will keep in the fridge for up to 2 weeks.

Nutrition per serving:
Calories 140 | Total carbohydrate 25 g | Sugars 14 g
Fat 3.5 g | Protein 3 g | Sodium 15 mg

Cherry and Greek yoghurt cake

Packed full of simple and complex carbohydrates, good fats from the nuts and seeds, and antioxidants from the fruit

We all know that cake and cycling go hand in hand, and this cake really is a cyclist's best friend. The acidity of the cherries, yoghurt and lemon gives this cake a lovely balance. The recipe would also work well with fresh or frozen blueberries.

Serves 12

100 g (3 ½ oz) rolled oats

100 g (3 ½ oz) ground almonds

50 g (2 oz) pistachio nuts

50 g (2 oz) chia seeds

80 g (3 oz) rice flour

1 teaspoon baking powder

½ teaspoon vanilla extract

100 g (3 ½ oz) unsalted butter, softened

140 ml good-quality maple syrup

zest of 1 lemon

250 ml (1 cup) full-fat Greek yoghurt

3 large free-range eggs, separated

300 g (11 oz) frozen or fresh cherries, stones removed

Nutrition per serving:

Calories 229 | Total carbohydrate 20 g | Sugars 9 g | Fat 14 g
Protein 6 g | Sodium 30 mg

1. Preheat the oven to 180°C/350°F/Gas 4.

2. Line a medium 22 cm x 22 cm (9 inch x 9 inch) cake tin with greaseproof paper.

3. In the bowl of a food processor, blitz the oats to a fine powder and transfer to a mixing bowl. Stir in the ground almonds, pistachio nuts, chia seeds, rice flour and baking powder; set aside.

4. In the bowl of the food processor blend the vanilla extract, butter, maple syrup, lemon zest, yoghurt and egg yolks.

5. In a separate bowl, whisk the egg whites until firm peaks form.

6. Fold the egg whites into the wet mix (butter/maple syrup) using a spatula, then fold this mix into the oat and nut mix. Finally, stir in the cherries and pour the mixture into the prepared cake tin.

7. Bake in the centre of the oven for 50–60 minutes. Allow to cool in the tin for 10 minutes and then transfer to a wire rack. Store in the fridge but bring up to room temperature before serving. Best eaten within a week.

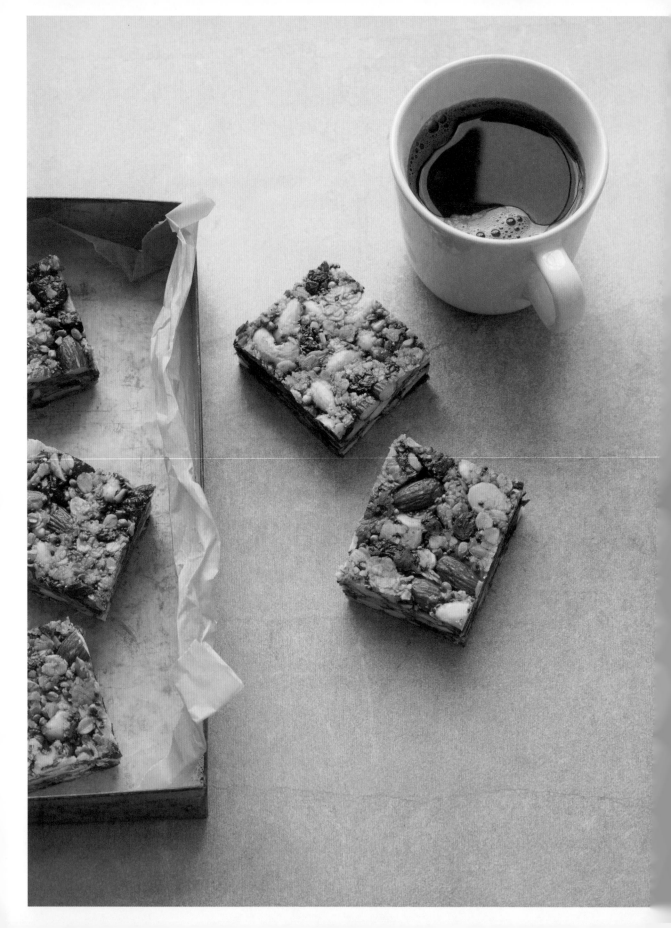

Fruit 'n' nut flapjacks

You can't beat a good flapjack for snacking, and these are perfect for on-the-bike refuelling too

These non-bake flapjacks have a really lovely texture due to the high ratio of nuts, seeds and dried fruit. This does make them highly calorific, though, so they are only for hard days out on the bike. You can use any mix of dried fruit that you fancy – the recipe works particular well with dried mixed citrus peel and a tablespoon of good-quality Seville orange marmalade.

Makes 24 x 60 g (2 ½ oz) flapjacks

100 g (3 ½ oz) almonds

100 g (3 ½ oz) hazelnuts

100 g (3 ½ oz) salted peanuts

100 g (3 ½ oz) cashew nuts

100 g (3 ½ oz) walnuts

50 g (2 oz) hemp seeds

50 g (2 oz) chia seeds

50 g (2 oz) sunflower seeds

50 g (2 oz) muscovado sugar

200 g (7 oz) honey

230 g (8 oz) unsalted butter

a pinch of Himalayan salt

250 g (9 oz) rolled oats

100 g (3 ½ oz) dried cherries

50 g (2 oz) raisins

50 g (2 oz) dried cranberries

50 g (2 oz) golden raisins

1. In a bowl, mix together all the nuts and seeds. Toast gently in a dry pan until golden brown (keep an eye on them as they will burn quickly) and set aside.

2. Place the sugar and honey in a saucepan and set over a medium heat to melt. Stir in the butter and salt; boil for 30 seconds.

3. Stir the nuts, seeds and the remaining ingredients together in the saucepan. Line a 22 cm x 22 cm (9 inch x 9 inch) baking tin with greaseproof paper and spray with a little olive oil. Press the mix into the tray and place in the fridge to set for 2–3 hours before slicing into 60 g (2 ½ oz) bars. Store in the fridge for a couple of weeks.

Nutrition per serving:

Calories 328 | Total carbohydrate 25 g | Sugars 14 g
Fat 23 g | Protein 7 g | Sodium 54 mg

Lemon polenta cake

Being naturally gluten free, this is ideal for after long rides when your stomach may be a little sensitive

OK, so this cake has a fair bit of butter and sugar, but it's very much a treat kind of cake. The polenta offers an interesting textural alternative to standard flour, and polenta is one of the most carbohydrate-dense grains on the planet. You can also serve this with some good-quality citrus yoghurt for an awesome dessert.

Serves 12

300 g (11 oz) butter, softened

300 g (11 oz) golden demerara sugar

zest and juice of 2 lemons (do not mix)

4 eggs, beaten

300 g (11 oz) ground almonds

150 g (5 oz) polenta

1 teaspoon baking powder

100 g (3 ½ oz) pistachio nuts

1 tablespoon poppy seeds

Nutrition per serving:

Calories 426 | Total carbohydrate 30 g | Sugars 20 g
Fat 30 g | Protein 9 g | Sodium 48 mg

1. Preheat the oven to 150°C/300°F/Gas 2. In the bowl of a mixer fitted with the paddle attachment, beat the butter, sugar and lemon zest for 4–5 minutes until creamy. Gradually incorporate the eggs, then the lemon juice.

2. Beat in the almonds, polenta and baking powder, then fold in the pistachio nuts and poppy seeds.

3. Line a 22 cm x 22 cm (9 inch x 9 inch) cake tin with greaseproof paper and spray with a little olive oil. Transfer the cake mix into the tin and bake for 60–70 minutes. This is quite a dense cake so it requires long, slow cooking. Allow to cool in the tin for 10 minutes and then transfer to a wire rack. Store in the fridge for up to a week.

Banana bread muffins

Not all muffin tops are bad! Perfect as a pick-me-up or breakfast on the go

Whether you make these as individual muffins or in a loaf tin, it's up to you. This is a really simple method and literally bomb-proof recipe!

Makes 8 good-sized muffins

3 ripe bananas, peeled

2 large free-range organic eggs

125 ml (½ cup) milk (either cow's milk or your favourite dairy-free alternative)

110 g (3 ½ oz) butter, melted

300 g (11 oz) gluten-free self-raising flour

110 g (3 ½ oz) brown sugar

1 tablespoon poppy seeds

2 teaspoons cinnamon

1 teaspoon each brown sugar and cinnamon, mixed for dusting

1 tablespoon flaked almonds

Nutrition per serving:

Calories 375 | Total carbohydrate 56 g | Sugars 20 g
Fat 15 g | Protein 6 g | Sodium 150 mg

1. Preheat the oven to 180°C/350°F/Gas 4. In the bowl of a food processor, blend the bananas to form a mash. Add the eggs, milk and melted butter, then gradually incorporate the flour, brown sugar, poppy seeds and cinnamon.

2. Use a 5 cm x 32 cm x 21.5 cm (2 inch x 12 inch x 8 inch) 6-cup muffin tray. You will need to cook these in two batches. Either line the muffin moulds with paper cases or spray with olive oil spray. Spoon the mixture into the muffin moulds and top with the brown sugar and cinnamon mix. Sprinkle over the flaked almonds.

3. Bake in the centre of the oven for 12–14 minutes until golden brown. Leave to cool in the tin for 5 minutes before transferring to a wire rack to cool completely. Store in an airtight container in the fridge. Best consumed within a week.

Courgette and orange muffins

Courgettes (zucchini) make a great base for cakes or muffins, and this is a fantastic way to get some veg in

As we all know, vegetables are good for us! Incorporating them into desserts and snacks adds to your veg count without even trying. Due to the demands we place on our bodies, cyclists should aim to exceed the traditionally recommended 'five a day'. In fact, double that. Courgettes are cheap to buy and even easier to grow at home, yet most people have no idea what to do with them. Here, the citrussy dried mixed peel and zest work really well with the neutral taste of the courgettes. But if you still don't fancy courgettes, this recipe works pretty well with grated carrot instead.

Makes 18 small muffins

3 eggs

2 large courgettes, grated

90 g (3 ½ oz) butter, melted

75 g (3 oz) maple syrup

75 g (3 oz) brown sugar

1 teaspoon vanilla extract

230 g (8 oz) ground almonds

140 g gluten-free oats

45 g (2 oz) raisins

45 g (2 oz) dried mixed peel

60 g (2 ½ oz) pecan nuts

1 tablespoon flax seeds

1 tablespoon chia seeds

1 teaspoon ground cinnamon

a pinch of sea salt

a pinch of freshly ground black pepper

grated zest of 2 oranges

1. Preheat the oven to 180°C/350°F/Gas 4.

2. Simply combine all the wet ingredients together in the bowl of a food mixer using the paddle attachment. Gradually add all the dry ingredients until well incorporated.

3. Use a 3 cm x 32 cm x 26 cm (1 inch x 12 inch x 10 inch) 12-cup muffin tray. Cook in two batches of eight to ensure even cooking. Either line the muffin moulds with paper cases or spray with olive oil spray. Spoon the mixture into muffin moulds and bake in the centre of the oven for 20–30 minutes until golden brown. Leave to cool in the tin for 5 minutes before transferring to a wire rack to cool completely. Store in an airtight container in the fridge. These are best consumed within a week.

Nutrition per serving:
Calories 238 | Total carbohydrate 18 g | Sugars 11 g
Fat 15 g | Protein 7 g | Sodium 35 mg

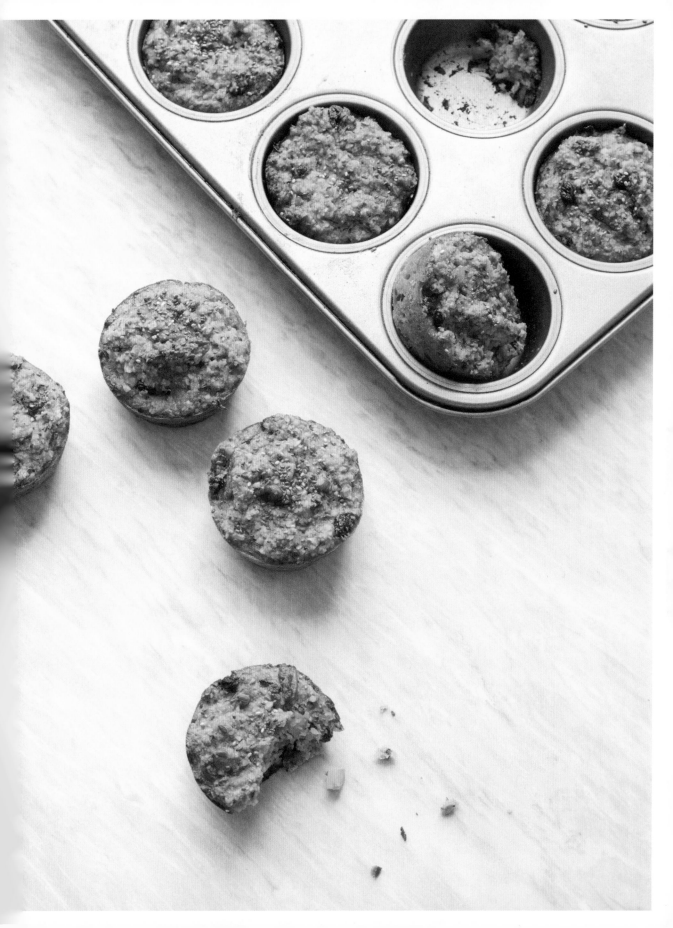

White chocolate and coconut bars

These may sound decadent, but they offer decent protein levels thanks to the nuts, protein powder and nut butter

This is an invention born out of a challenge. Lee, a training buddy of mine, asked me to make a protein bar recipe that actually works after having countless disasters trying to make his own. The aim was to create that sweet and salty combo which we crave after hard training sessions or long rides, to restock those glycogen and electrolyte stores and help repair tired muscles. This is the result and I think you'll agree it tastes like a real treat.

Makes 15 x 50 g bars

230 g (8 oz) gluten-free oats

50 g (2 oz) dried coconut

1 teaspoon Himalayan salt

30 g (1 oz) goji berries

100 g (3 ½ oz) dried mango, chopped

100 g (3 ½ oz) dried cherries, chopped

100 g (3 ½ oz) cashew nuts

16 g (½ oz) chia seeds

125 ml (½ cup) milk

75 g (3 oz) vanilla protein powder

2 tablespoons runny honey

80 g (3 oz) white chocolate

60 g (2 ½ oz) coconut oil

80 g (3 oz) peanut butter

1. In a bowl, mix together all the dry ingredients and set aside.

2. Whisk together the milk, vanilla protein powder and runny honey in another bowl until you have a smooth paste.

3. In a saucepan set over a low heat, melt the white chocolate and coconut oil together, then stir in the peanut butter.

4. In a large mixing bowl, combine the milk mix with the white chocolate mix, then stir in all the dry ingredients. Line a shallow 22 cm x 22 cm (9 inch x 9 inch) baking tin with greaseproof paper and spray with olive oil, then press the mixture into the tin. Place in the fridge for 60–90 minutes to firm up before slicing into 50 g (2 oz) bars.

Nutrition per serving:

Calories 257 | Total carbohydrate 32 g | Sugars 16 g
Fat 10 g | Protein 8.5 g | Sodium 118 mg

Easy-peasy chocolate protein mousse

An easy-to-make chocolate dessert that is high in protein, perfect for overnight recovery

This is a really nostalgic milk-based pudding combining really good quality chocolate, extra protein from the protein powder, seeds and nuts, and naturally sweet honey. There's no bad news here!

Serves 2

120 ml (½ cup) coconut milk

1 tablespoon honey

60 g (2 ½ oz) chocolate protein powder

1 teaspoon cocoa nibs (Grue de Cacao)

1 tablespoon cocoa powder

1 tablespoon desiccated coconut

1 teaspoon chia seeds

1 tablespoon chopped cashews

chopped banana or fresh cherries, to serve

1. In the bowl of a food processor blend the coconut milk, honey, protein powder, cocoa nibs and cocoa powder. Stir in the coconut, chia seeds and cashews.

2. Spoon the mixture into a couple of ramekins and then place in the fridge for 30 minutes to firm up. Serve with chopped banana or fresh cherries on the side.

Nutrition per serving:
Calories 288 | Total carbohydrate 18 g | Sugars 12 g
Fat 13 g | Protein 26 g | Sodium 4 mg

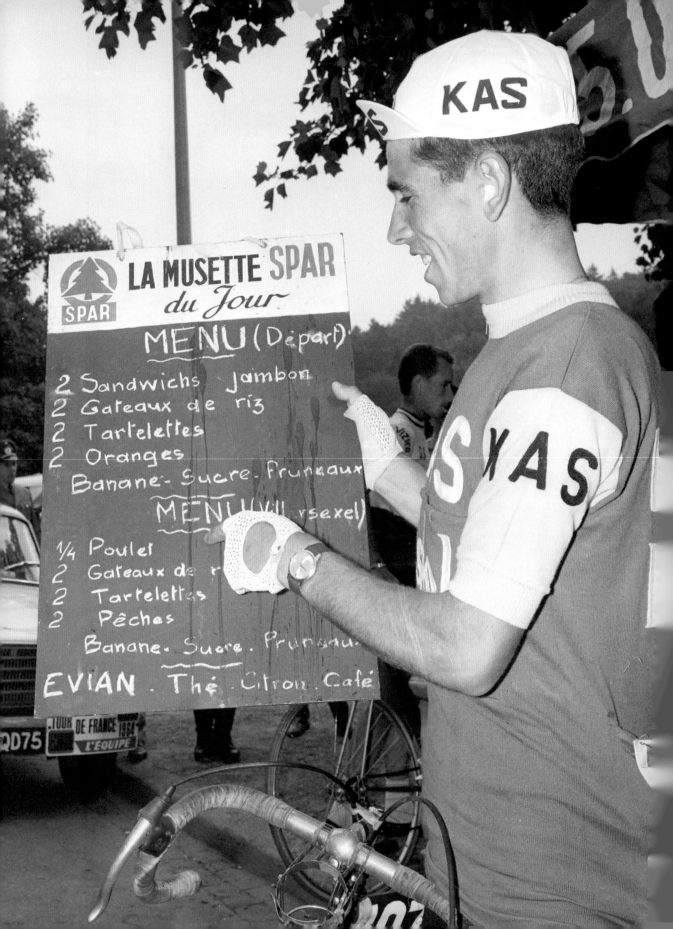

Nutritional Plans

Following a nutritional plan will
enable you to make sure your fuelling
matches your training programme and
that you have sufficient levels of all the
nutrients your body needs.

Training, eating, sleeping… hopefully, these
aren't the only components in your life, but
they are the ones that will improve your cycling
performance. Your diet is an essential and
integral part of your training and racing– not
only is it fuel for each exertion, but it prepares
the body for exercise and completes the effort
that you put in: following a nutritional plan is
every bit as important as sticking to your
training plan.

Spanish rider Joaquim Galera reviews a
Tour de France stage menu. While it is
important to keep to a nutritional plan,
give yourself a night off every now and
then. It'll help you sustain the plan in
the long run.

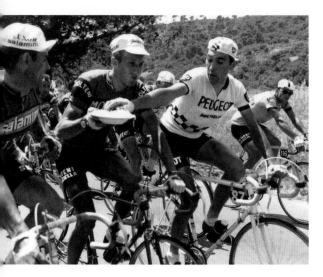

The size of portions will vary massively from rider to rider, but start from the 60-20-20 (carbohydrate-protein-fat) guidelines and you really can't go far wrong. Here Belgian cycling legend Eddy Merckx helps himself to pasta from Italian rider Gianni Motta, during the 1957 Giro d'Italia.

Performance cyclists can expect to be undertaking two moderate distance sessions during the week and one or two longer-distance rides at the weekend depending on race commitments. Rest days are essential and there may also be gym, turbo or weight training sessions to fit in. Any nutritional plan will shadow this work, allowing for pre-ride and recovery meals on tough days and maintaining weight and health on light training and rest days.

Most cyclists also have a cycle of pre-season training, race season, post-season rest (I suggest athletes give themselves a complete break for a couple of weeks) and off-season preparation. Meals and portions will vary from season to season accordingly. The carbohydrate-heavy meals of race season and periods of hard training will not be appropriate off-season and during base training you might switch to a higher protein ratio as you seek to lose weight or build endurance. You should therefore be making your plan in weekly blocks. This allows for changes to your schedule and for you to shop effectively – you should be able to get all you need from a weekly shop and a midweek top-up of fresh produce. Plan what you will eat in all main meals, but remember to buy any ad-hoc and on-the-bike snacks you may need (*see also* p. 154). Variety is key here, both in motivating you to sustain the diet and ensuring all bases are covered in terms of nutrients. The size of portions will vary massively from rider to rider, but start from the 60-20-20 (carbohydrate-protein-fat) guidelines and you really can't go far wrong.

It's your performance; it's your responsibility. This applies to sticking to your plan and adjusting your intake to suit your own body.

I suggest you keep a diary of exercise, food and sleep, annotating it with how you feel, physically and mentally. This will enable you to work out your optimum diet through trial and error. Always make sure you test out new foods in training, and don't risk disaster by trying something new on race day. Apps such as MyFitnessPal (www.myfitnesspal.com) and TrainingPeaks (www.trainingpeaks.com) can help you match calorie intake to your training schedule and ensure you do not put on weight. However, if you do wish to lose weight then you need to maintain a balanced meal plan with a calorie deficit. It is almost impossible to have a large calorie deficit and still perform high-intensity sessions on the bike, but a 10 per cent calorie deficit a day at certain times in your yearly training cycle will enable you to lose weight and train effectively.

Oh, and one final thing: give yourself a night off every now and then – even once a week, if you want. It'll help you sustain the plan in the long run. If Olympic cyclists and Grand Tour riders do it, so can you. The odd steak and chips, a kebab, a dirty burger – whatever you fantasise about eating as you grind out a gruelling 50-mile ride home – isn't going to ruin anything, I promise.

I suggest you keep a diary of exercise, food and sleep, annotating it with how you feel, physically and mentally. This will enable you to work out your optimum diet through trial and error.

Sample Race Day Nutritional Plan

	Pre-race Day (Friday)	Race Day (Morning Race)	Race Day (Afternoon Race)	Race Day (Evening Race)
Breakfast	Classic bircher (*see* p.64)	Piña colada bircher (*see* p.66)	Poached eggs on toast	Multiseed pancakes (*see* p. 46)
		Make up the night before to save time.	Eat as soon as you get up.	Eat as soon as you get up.
		Optimally, eat three hours before start time.	Add avocado if you are feeling hungry.	Serve with your choice of sweet or savoury toppings.
Snack	Budgie cage bar (*see* p. 170)	Nutty slack (*see* p. 148)		
		Post-race		
		Within 30 minutes of finishing.		
Lunch	BBQ spiced chicken with quinoa (*see* p. 126)	BBQ spiced chicken with quinoa (*see* p. 126)	Piña colada bircher (*see* p. 66)	BBQ spiced chicken with quinoa (*see* p. 126)
		Make up double quantities the day before.	Optimally, eat three hours before start time.	Make up double quantities the day before.
Snack	Nitrate turbo booster (*see* p. 150)			Mia's cherry go-go (*see* p. 168)
				or
				Piña colada bircher (*see* p. 66)
				Optimally, three hours before start time
Dinner	'Scottish' paella (*see* p. 102)	Turkey mince chilli (*see* p. 86)	Turkey mince chilli (*see* p. 86)	Hookers' pasta (*see* p. 94)
		Make up in advance.	Make up in advance.	Simple carbs for glycogen replenishment.
		Serve with baked sweet potato or brown rice.	Serve with baked sweet potato or brown rice.	Quick and easy to cook from scratch.
Pre-bed	Banana bread muffin (*see* p. 177)	Easy-peasy chocolate protein mousse (*see* p. 181)	Easy-peasy chocolate protein mousse (*see* p. 181)	Easy-peasy chocolate protein mousse (*see* p. 181)

Sample Weekly Nutritional Plan

	Sunday *(Long Ride – Afternoon)*	Monday *(Rest Day)*	Tuesday *(Intervals – Evening)*	Wednesday *(Gym/Turbo)*	Thursday *(Light Ride)*
Breakfast	Kedgeree (*see* p. 60)	Piña colada bircher (*see* p. 66)	Multiseed pancakes (*see* p. 46)	Classic apple and cinnamon bircher (*see* p. 67)	Huevos rancheros (*see* p. 133)
Snack	Lemon polenta cake (*see* p. 176)		Lemon polenta cake (*see* p. 176)	Lemon polenta cake (*see* p. 176)	
Lunch	Beetroot and blueberry bircher (*see* p. 68)	Grandmother's chicken soup (*see* p. 76)	Chicken and avocado Caesar salad (*see* p. 118)	Avocado coleslaw with greens and cold smoked salmon (*see* p. 120)	Greek yoghurt with avocado, green pepper, coriander and mango (*see* p. 124)
			Optimally, eat three hours before start time		
Snack	Nitrate turbo booster (*see* p. 150)	Handful of nuts and dried fruit	Mocha bircher (*see* p. 65)	Supergreens smoothie (*see* p. 151)	Courgette and orange muffin (*see* p. 178)
				Optimally, eat three hours before start time.	
Dinner	'Scottish' paella (*see* p. 102)	Sesame and soy tuna niçoise (*see* p. 114)	Chicken sausages with spicy bean cassoulet and crispy polenta (*see* p. 90)	Smoked mackerel with watercress salad, beetroot and grainy mustard new potatoes (*see* p. 122)	Asian-style turkey burgers (*see* p. 104)
			Make up in advance		
			Tropical rice pudding (*see* p. 166)	Baked figs with quark (*see* p. 167)	

Acknowledgements

After stepping out of a Michelin-starred kitchen it took me a little time to find 'what next'. This transition would not have been possible without some awesome people who have hassled, trusted and advised me in many ways.

Over the years many people have said 'you should do a book' – in reality having the food knowledge is the easiest part of the whole process, so I need to say a huge thank you to a number of good people who have helped me out.

There is always a spark for any idea – we had an initial brain dump for the Performance Chef business in 2014 with Gwen Jorgensen and Pat Lemieux, and their open-minded approach to optimising performance was the kick-start I needed to get into cooking great food for athletes. Gwen always says you need to 'focus on the process not the outcome'. Food and nutrition play a huge part in the process. Pat is my culinary padawan.

My partner Vicky is the one who keeps the admin side of my life in order, and quite frankly this book would not have happened without her. Deadlines are there to be pushed, right? Vicky is also head hydro ceramic technician (washer up) at home but she does get fed like a princess in return.

For their honest and forthright views on new recipes, thanks to the kids – Megan, Kyle and my 'little' girls, Freya and Mia. I have also plagiarised Freya's muffin recipe and Mia's cherry balls for my own benefit.

Bike coach Matt Bottrill gave me the opportunity to work with ambitious, talented and focused amateur cyclists when he was starting his own business, and he quickly recognised the benefits of aligning quality training and real food with common sense nutritional advice. Rich Gambo, Lee Morgan, Simon Beldon and John Dewey were some of my initial test pilots, and I owe them a big thank you.

I get a huge buzz from working with world class cyclists on a regular basis; they give me invaluable feedback and trust me to feed them when it really matters. To Hayley Simmonds, Alex Dowsett, Dan Bigham, Katie Archibald, Charlie Tanfield, Ethan Hayter, Callum Skinner and Steve Bate: keep that chain tight and never stop pushing.

To be able to constantly develop new recipes and eat them all, I need to ride and race my bikes a lot. I am hugely fortunate to have the support of Specialized UK, Will and DA. Thanks also to Simon and Natalie at Drag2Zero – they give me the very best bikes, kit and advice out there!

In the kitchen, I use Miele equipment. It is simply the best you can get for domestic cooking, and allows a level of consistency and precision that means my recipes work time and time again. Nerdy food science is not my thing, so I'm lucky I can call on Dr Jamie Pringle and Kathryn Brown for a level of understanding that quite frankly is way beyond a 'thick chef'.

I also have to thank Lee Hemani, who has always given me great honest business advice and been a bloody good mate when the chips were down.

'Patience is a virtue' must be the team motto at Bloomsbury Sport, who brought the whole book to life! I truly appreciate the saint-like attributes of Matt Lowing in particular. And for a stunning finished product, thanks to Adrian Besley, Allie Collins, photographers Clare Winfield and Grant Pritchard, food stylist Rebecca Woods and designer Sian Rance, plus Lizzy Ewer,

Katherine Macpherson, Alice Graham and everyone else at Bloomsbury.

This project has probably aged Adam Ackworth, my agent – he looks after the odd feral chef and normally does deals for elite athletes. Chefs are much harder work apparently!

Lastly, a huge thanks to all the food fans and cyclists who regularly comment on the food I cook. We are only just getting started.

About the Author

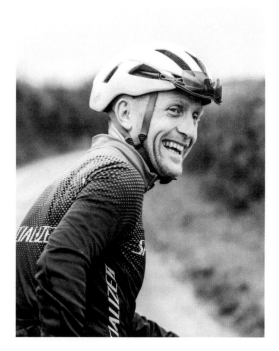

Alan Murchison is a Michelin-starred chef with over 25 years' experience working in starred restaurants (he held a Michelin star for over a decade and had 4 AA Rosettes whist Executive Chef at L'Ortolan restaurant in Berkshire), he is also a multiple World and European age group duathlon champion, national level master's cyclist and ex-international endurance runner.

Alan provides bespoke nutritional support for athletes across a number of sports, although predominantly for cyclists. He is a consultant with British Cycling and works with athletes across a range of abilities, from first-timers looking to just complete an event to current Olympic gold medallists.

@performance.chef

Index